Dosage Calculations
Demystified

Demystified Series

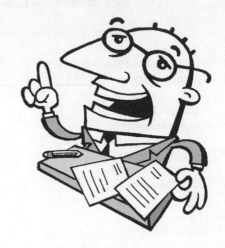

Dosage Calculations Demystified

Jim Keogh

New York   Chicago   San Francisco   Lisbon   London
Madrid   Mexico City   Milan   New Delhi   San Juan
Seoul   Singapore   Sydney   Toronto

The McGraw·Hill Companies

Library of Congress Cataloging-in-Publication Data

Keogh, James Edward, date.
    Dosage calculations demystified / Jim Keogh.
        p.   ;   cm. — (DeMYSTiFied)
    Includes index.
    ISBN 978-0-07-160284-6 (alk. paper)   .
    1.   Pharmaceutical arithmetic.   I. Title. II. Series: McGraw-Hill "Demystified" series.
    [DNLM: 1. Drug Dosage Calculations. 2. Drug Therapy—nursing. 3. Medication Errors—prevention & control. 4.   Prescriptions, Drug.   QV 748 K37d 2009]
    RS57.K46 2009
    615'.1401513—dc22

                                                                                    2008037712

McGraw-Hill books are available at special quantity discounts to use as premiums and sales promotions, or for use in corporate training programs. To contact a special sales representative, please visit the Contact Us page at www.mhprofessional.com.

1 2 3 4 5 6 7 8 9 0   DOC/DOC   0 1 4 3 2 1 0 9 8

ISBN 978-0-07-160284-6
MHID 0-07-160284-4

Sponsoring Editor
  Judy Bass

Editorial Supervisor
  David E. Fogarty

Project Manager
  Harleen Chopra, International Typesetting
  and Composition

Copy Editor
  Ragini Pandey, International Typesetting and
  Composition

Proofreader
  Manish Tiwari, International Typesetting and
  Composition

Indexer
  Broccoli Information Management

Production Supervisor
  Pamela A. Pelton

Composition
  International Typesetting and Composition

Art Director, Cover
  Jeff Weeks

Printed and bound by RR Donnelley.

This book is dedicated to Anne, Sandy, Joanne, Amber-Leigh Christine, and Shawn, without whose help and support this book couldn't have been written.

ABOUT THE AUTHOR

Jim Keogh, RN, is a member of the faculty at both New York University and Saint Peter's College in New Jersey. He is a graduate nurse and is the coauthor of *Medical-Surgical Nursing Demystified, Pharmacology Demystified, Medical Billing and Coding Demystified, Nurse Management Demystified, Medical Charting Demystified,* and several other books.

CONTENTS AT A GLANCE

CONTENTS

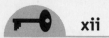

Contents

PREFACE

Calculating the correct dose to administer to the patient is challenging unless you follow a proven approach that is used in *Dosage Calculations Demystified*. Topics are presented in an order in which many nurses and nursing students like to learn them—starting with the basics and then gradually moving on to techniques used in our nation's leading medical facilities every day to ensure patients receive the proper dose of medication.

Each chapter follows a time-tested formula that first explains techniques in an easy-to-read style and then shows how you can use it in the real-world healthcare environment. You can then test your knowledge at the end of each chapter to be sure that you have mastered nurse management skills. There is little room for you to go adrift.

CHAPTER 1: MEDICATION ORDER AND MEDICATION

A critical aspect of the nurse's job is to read and understand a medication order and then calculate the dose based on the medication on hand. You might be wondering why you must calculate the dose when the dose is specified in the medication order. The dose in the medication order is the dose of the medicine that the patient is receiving. The calculated dose is the dose of the medicine on hand that is given to the patient to equal the dose in the medication order.

Before learning how to calculate a dose, you'll need to understand how to read a medication order and medication labels, which is covered in this chapter.

CHAPTER 2: THE FORMULA METHOD

Based on the medical diagnosis, the physician prescribes a dose of the medication that will improve the patient's condition. Sometimes this is the same dose that appears on the medication label, which means that the patient receives the complete content of the container.

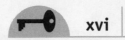
However, the medication might be a different dose and thus requires the nurse to calculate the amount of medication to administer to the patient.

Two methods are used to calculate the dose. These are the formula method and the proportion method. Both methods arrive at the same dose. You'll learn the formula method in this chapter.

CHAPTER 3: THE RATIO-PROPORTION METHOD

The goal of the ratio-proportion method is to solve for X using a simple algebraic expression X in the dose. Other elements of the expression are given in the medication order and on the medication label. You'll learn how to use the ratio-proportion method in this chapter and be in the position to choose the ratio-proportion method or the formula method to calculate the dose of medication for your patients.

CHAPTER 4: INTRAVENOUS CALCULATIONS

Your patient may require intravenous therapy. How much medication the patient receives depends on the rate of flow of the I.V. The rate is controlled by setting the number of drops of fluid that is administered to the patient each minute. Alternatively, the rate is controlled by the number of milliliters delivered each hour to the patient by a medication pump.

The medication order specifies the medication, the volume, and the time period within which the medication is infused into the patient. You calculate the number of drops or the milliliters setting for the medication pump. You'll learn how to perform these calculations in this chapter.

CHAPTER 5: CALCULATING PEDIATRIC DOSES

The dose of medication for a pediatric patient must be carefully calculated based on the patient's weight because even a small discrepancy can endanger the youngster's health. Furthermore, there is a limited amount of any medication that the pediatric patient should receive within 24 hours. Before administrating medication, you'll need to determine the total amount of the medication the youngster has already received and then calculate the dose using the patient's weight. You'll learn how to perform both calculations in this chapter.

CHAPTER 6: CALCULATING A HEPARIN DOSE

Heparin is an anticoagulant (prevents the formation of blood clots) and is administered as a subcutaneous (S.C.) injection or administered in an I.V. and is also used to flush a Hep-Lock that connects I.V. tubing to the patient's vein.

So far nearly all dosages that you calculated throughout this book used metric units—milligrams, micrograms, and milliliters. Heparin is different and is measured in USP units (U), which is a standard set by the United States Pharmacopeial Convention Inc. In this chapter you'll learn how to read a medication order for heparin and calculate the proper dose to administer to your patient.

CHAPTER 7: CALCULATING A DOPAMINE DOSE

Dopamine is a neurotransmitter formed in the brain that affects movement, emotion, and perception. Calculating the proper dose of dopamine to administer to your patient is a little different from the way you calculated the dose of other medications because the prescribed dose is per kilogram and the medication on hand is a concentration. A concentration is a mixture of I.V. fluid that contains a specific amount of dopamine.

Before you calculate the dose for your patient, you must use the prescribed dose to calculate prescribed dose for your patient's weight and you also need to calculate the amount of dopamine in a milliliter of the concentration. You'll learn these calculations in this chapter.

CHAPTER 8: CALCULATING A DOSE FOR CHILDREN USING BODY SURFACE AREA

Weight-based dose calculations determine the proper dose based on the patient's weight. Some physicians prefer body surface area rather than weight as the basis for calculating the dose. Body surface area reflects both weight and height and is considered to be the most accurate way to calculate a dose for a child because it considers two measurement of a child. In this chapter you'll learn how to calculate the proper dose of medication for your young patient by using the child's body surface area.

CHAPTER 9: ENTERAL TUBE FEEDING

Patients who have a stroke, tracheoesophageal fistula, esophageal atresia, and other conditions that affect swallowing are a risk for aspiration pneumonia and malnutrition. Physicians take the preemptive strategy of placing the patient on enteral tube feeding (feeding the patient using a tube inserted into the gastrointestinal tract), which greatly reduces the risk for aspiration and assures that nutrients reach the stomach.

Enteral tube feedings usually come in full strength; however, the physician typically orders enteral tube feedings at less than full strength. This requires you to dilute the enteral tube feeding before it is administered to your patient. In this

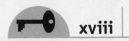

chapter you'll learn how to calculate the fraction or percentage of dilution that must be applied to the full concentration of the enteral tube feeding.

APPENDIX A: ANSWERING TRICKY QUESTIONS

All dose calculation questions that you'll be asked on a test can be solved using formulas learned in this book or by using basic math that you learned in grammar school. However, some questions are purposely written to confuse you. In this chapter, you'll see tricky questions that are similar to those that you find on tests and you'll learn ways of solving those questions.

APPENDIX B: QUICK REFERENCE

Right before a test you probably want to refresh what you've learned through this book. The "Quick Reference" is the only place you need to look. There you'll find a summary of all the formulas and other key information needed to pass your dose calculation test.

ACKNOWLEDGMENT

I am very thankful to Rebecca Rigolosi who painstakingly technically reviewed this book.

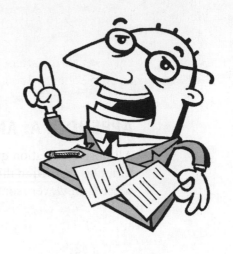

Dosage Calculations
Demystified

CHAPTER 1

Medication Order and Medication

Giving a patient medication isn't as simple as placing a tablet in the patient's hand and asking him to swallow it. It must be the right medication and dose and administered according to the physician's order.

A critical aspect of the nurse's job is to read and understand a medication order and then calculate the dose based on the medication on hand. You might be wondering why you must calculate the dose when the dose is specified in the medication order. The dose in the medication order is the dose of the medicine that the patient is receiving. The calculated dose is the dose of the medicine on hand that is given to the patient to equal the dose in the medication order. Sounds confusing? This will be crystal clear after you finish the next chapter.

Before learning how to calculate a dose, you'll need to understand how to read a medication order and medication labels, which is covered in this chapter.

Learning Objectives

➤ Medication order

➤ Medication record

➤ Taking off orders

➤ Avoid common errors when using the MAR type of charting systems

➤ Medication labels

Key Words

JCAHO

Joint Commission on Accreditation of Healthcare Organizations

MAR

Medication administration

Medication Administration Record

Medication dose

Medication name

Medication order date and time

Medication order renewal

Medication route

Medication strength

Military time

Patient identification

PRN medication orders

Sign

Symptom

Medication Order

When a patient complains about aches, pains, and other symptoms (subjective), the physician assesses the patient for objective data called **signs** that lead to a medical diagnosis and treatment plan. Although the term physician is used throughout this book, other healthcare professionals such as nurse practitioners, midwives, and physician's assistants can make a medical diagnosis and prescribe medication.

For example, the patient complains about a sore throat (**symptom**). Upon examination the physician notices red and swollen tonsils, white patches on the patient's throat, swollen lymph glands in the neck, and a temperature of 101°F (signs) that might lead to the medical diagnosis of strep throat.

Medication is prescribed as part of the treatment plan for many medical diagnoses. The prescription is a **medication order** that is sometimes referred to as a doctor's order. All medication orders are written—hand written—or entered into a computerized order system.

Figure 1.1   Is this 20 or 2U?

Figure 1.1 looks like a 20 but really is 2 U. The handwritten U is poorly written. However, the error is easily detected by the nurse because if the value of the dose is 20, as it can be interpreted, then the medication order is missing the unit of measurement for the value and therefore isn't a valid medication order.

A similar problem occurs with the abbreviation for international units, which is IU. A poorly written U can be misread as a V resulting the abbreviation being read as IV instead of IU. And this too can be caught because the medication order would be missing the unit of measurement.

The **Joint Commission on Accreditation of Healthcare Organizations (JCAHO)** developed a list of abbreviations that should not be used, which are illustrated in Table 1.1. Some healthcare facilities have policies that add to this do-not-use list of abbreviations and instead require physicians to write out the complete word.

Another common error occurs with decimal values. It is easy to miss the decimal point. For example, .2 mg could be misread as 2 mg or 5.0 mg can be misinterpreted as 50 mg. Physician must use a leading zero for decimal values such as 0.2 mg and drop values and exclude the decimal point and zero if no decimal value is used such as 5 mg.

Table 1.1   Do Not Use Abbreviations

Don't Use	Use in Place	Problem
U	Unit	Misread for zero
IV	International Units	Misread for IV for 10
Q.D., QD, q.d., qd	Daily	Confusing to read
Q.O.D., QOD, q.o.d., qod	Every other day	Confusing to read
.X mg	0.X mg	Decimal point overlooked
X.0 mg	X mg	Decimal point overlooked
MS	Morphine sulfate	Can be confused with magnesium sulfate
MSO_4	Morphine sulfate	Can be confused with magnesium sulfate ($MgSO_4$)
$MgSO_4$	Magnesium sulfate	Can be confused with morphine sulfate (MSO_4)

Table 1.2   Abbreviations for Medication Administration Routes

Abbreviation	Route
P.O.	By mouth
I.D.	Intradermal
I.M.	Intramuscular
I.V.	Intravenous
S.C.	Subcutaneous
T.D.	Transdermal

Medication Route

The physician must specify the way the medication is to be administered to the patient, which is referred to as the route. The route is typically identified by the common abbreviations in Table 1.2

Medication Administration Time and Frequency

The physician prescribes the time and frequency drug administration based on a number of factors including absorption, side effects, interactions with other medication, and the desired effect of the drug on the patient.

The time when the medication is given to the patient is usually at fixed hours according to the healthcare facilities policy such as 6 p.m. meds. Sometimes physicians will prescribe a specific time to administer the medication, but many times the frequency is specified and the nurse determines the actual time based on the healthcare facility's policy.

Table 1.3 contains abbreviations that are used to specify the frequency of when to administer medication.

Signature

The signature of the physician must be legible on the medication order otherwise the medication order is invalid. In addition, some physicians such as those in training or whose authority is limited by the healthcare facility may require a cosignature of another physician to validate the medication order.

Typically an attending physician must cosign medication orders written by interns and residents.

PRN Medication Orders

A **PRN medication order** directs the nurse to administer the medication as needed by the patient and should provide instructions to the nurse as to when to give the

Table 1.3 Frequencies of Administering Medication and Abbreviations

Abbreviation	Frequency
$\bar{a}$	Before
a.c.	Before meals
b.i.d. or bid	Twice a day
b.i.w.	Twice a week
h or hr	hour
h.s.	Hour of sleep or at bedtime
min	minute
noc or noct	At night
o.n.	Every night
$\bar{p}$	after
p.c.	After meals
q.	Every or each
q.a.m.	Every morning
q.h. or qh	Every hour
qXh	Every X hour where X is the number of hours
qhs or q.h.s.	Every night at bedtime
q.i.d. or qid	Four times a day
Stat or STAT	Immediately or at once
t.i.d. or tid	Three times a day
t.i.w.	Three times a week
PRN	As needed

medication. The instructions typically specify a sign or symptom such as a blood pressure reading, temperature, or if the patient reports pain.

The physician must specify the patient and date and time the medication order, name the medication, dose, and route and sign the order. Without any of these, the medication order is invalid.

MEDICATION ORDER RENEWAL

Although the physician determines when to discontinue a medication order based on the patient's condition, healthcare facilities have a **medication order renewal** policy that requires certain medication orders automatically discontinued after a

Table 1.4   Examples of When Medication Orders Are Automatically Discontinued

Medication	Discontinued
PRN-controlled medication	72 hours
Anticoagulants	24 hours 14 days, if the physician specifies the duration of the treatment
Antibiotics	10 days
Antineoplastic	24 hours 7 days, if the physician specifies the duration of the treatment
Parenteral nutrition	4 days
Schedule II medication (high potential for abuse)	72 hours 7 days, if the physician specifies the duration of the treatment
Schedule III (Moderate physical dependency)	7 days
Schedule IV (limited physical dependency)	7 days
Schedule V (log potential for abuse)	7 days

specified period of time. The physician must write a new medication order if the medication is to be continued.

A common practice is to have all medication orders discontinued after 14 days. There are exceptions, which are shown in Table 1.4.

The Medication Record

The Medication Administration Record is used to schedule when patients are to receive medication and record when the medication is administered and who administered it.

The design of a MAR differs among healthcare facilities; however, each has the same sections. These are

- Patient Information (Figure 1.2): This includes the patient's name, identification number, room number, diagnosis, and allergies.
- Schedule Medications (Figure 1.3): These are medications that are given regularly to the patient to maintain a therapeutic level such as once a day for seven days.

Unit	Patient's Name	Allergies	Primary Nurse
Med Surg	Susan Jones	None	Bob Marks
Room #			**Social Worker**
1601		**Age**	Roberta Johnson
		52	**Resident Physician**
		DOB	Dr. Anne Ford
		03/05/55	**Attending Physician**
			Dr. John Merk

Figure 1.2 Patient Information includes information that identifies the patient.

Medication Administration Record

Order Date Initials	Exp. Date Time	Medication - Dosage - Frequency Rt. Of Adm.	HR	4/1	4/2	4/3	4/4	4/5	4/6	4/7

Figure 1.3 Regularly scheduled medications are listed in Schedule Medications.

- Single Orders (Figure 1.4): These are medications that are administered once for an immediate effect such as epinephrine given STAT for anaphylactic shock.

- PRN Medications (Figure 1.5): These are medications given as needed such as NSAID for pain relief.

- Signature (Figure 1.6): Each healthcare provider who administers medication to the patient must be identified by full signature, title, and initials entered into the signature section of the MAR. Initials are then placed on the MAR alongside the medications that the healthcare provider administered to the patient.

Code		
O = Omitted	/ = Outdated	Cut = Discontinued
1 = Upper Outer Quadrant R Buttock	7 = Rt. Lateral Thigh	13 = Lt. Anterior Lateral Abdomen
2 = Upper Outer Quadrant L Buttock	8 = Lt. Lateral Thigh	14 = Rt. Posterior Lateral Abdomen
3 = Rt. Deltoid	9 = Rt. Ventrogluteal Area	15 = Lt. Posterior Lateral Abdomen
4 = Lt. Deltoid	10 = Lt. Ventrogluteal Area	16 = Rt. Upper Outer Arm
5 = Rt. Mid Anterior Thigh	11 = Abdomen	17 = Lt. Upper Outer Arm
6 = Lt. Mid Anterior Thigh	12 = Rt. Anterior Lateral Abdomen	

Single Orders - Pre-Operatives Stat-Meds						
Order Date Initials	Medication - Dosage - Route	Date Time	Adm. Time	Time Given	Site	Nurse Initial

Figure 1.4 Medications that are administered not on a schedule are listed in Single Orders.

PRN Medications								
Order Date Initials	Stop Date	Medication - Dosage - Frequency Rt. Of Adm.	PRN Medication s- Doses Given					
			Date					
			Time					
			Init.					
			Site					
			Date					
			Time					
			Init.					
			Site					
			Date					
			Time					
			Init.					
			Site					

Figure 1.5 Medications that are given at the request of the patient are listed in PRN Medications

Full Signature	Title	Initial
Bob Marks	RN	BM
Mary Adams	RN	MA

Figure 1.6 The Signature section contains the signature and corresponding initials of the nurse who administered medication to the patient.

CREATING A NEW MAR

A new MAR is created when the patient is admitted to the healthcare facility by the admissions staff or by the unit secretary who enters general information about the patient on the MAR, and places it into the MAR section of the patient's chart.

Prescriptions, written by a physician for medication, are copied from the Medical Orders section of the patient's chart and entered into the appropriate section of the MAR using a process called *taking off orders* (see "Taking Off Orders").

A licensed RN is responsible for taking off orders although some healthcare facilities permit the unit secretary to take off orders, if reviewed and signed off by the patient's primary nurse. The patient's primary nurse is legally responsible for the accuracy in the transcribing of medical orders on the MAR.

INFORMATION ABOUT MEDICATIONS

The MAR is a time-saving tool because it contains information needed to administer medications to a patient, except for orders that are cancelled or have not been taken off as yet. It is for this reason that you must always review the latest medical orders prior to administering any medication.

For each medication, the MAR contains

- Order Date: This is the date that the physician ordered the medication.
- Expiration Date: The order is no longer valid on or after the expiration date.
- Medication Name: This is usually the brand name of the medication.
- Dose: The amount of the medication the patient receives.
- Frequency: The number of doses the patient receives.
- Route of Administration: The route in which the medication is given to the patient.
- Site of Administration: Where was the medication administered if medication was administered in an injection?
- Date and Time: The day and hour that the medication must be administered.

USING THE MAR

At the beginning of each shift, the primary nurse reviews the MAR and identifies medications scheduled to be administered to the patient during the shift. The primary nurse also reviews the patient's chart for any new orders or cancelled orders that were written since the MAR was last updated. These orders if they exist are then taken off by the primary nurse.

HINT *Make a note of orders that are scheduled to expire at the end of the shift. Depending on the patient's condition and the nature of the order, you may want to ask the physician if the order should be renewed.*

Next, each medication is located on the unit. Medications delivered regularly by the pharmacy are usually placed in the patient's drawer in the medical cabinet or in the medication room. Each is labeled with the patient's name, identification, and room number. It is important to locate medications at the beginning of the shift thus allowing time to follow up with the pharmacy if the medication can't be found.

Before preparing to administer medication, one last check is made of the Medical Order section of the patient's chart to determine if the physician cancelled the order or prescribed new medication. This is an important step since in a busy unit, the primary nurse may not have the opportunity to speak directly with the physician.

The MAR is updated once the medication is administered to the patient. Some healthcare facilities require the primary nurse to take the MAR into the patient's room when administering medication so the MAR can be immediately updated giving little room for error.

Other healthcare facilities require the primary nurse to update the MAR immediately upon returning to the nurse's station after administering the medication to the patient. This leaves room for error since the primary nurse can easily be distracted and fail to remember to update the MAR.

The MAR is updated using one of three methods depending on the order:

- Scheduled medication: Write your initials in the cells that corresponds to the date and time that the medication was ordered.

- Single Orders: Write the date, time, site, and your initials.

- PRN: Enter the date, time, site, and your initials.

CAUTION *Never update the MAR before administering medication.*

Taking Off Orders

Medication orders must be copied from the Medical Orders section of the patient's chart to the MAR. This process is called taking off order. This is a critical process because failure to accurately transfer the order can have serious consequences for the patient.

Many healthcare facilities require a RN to take off orders, however some healthcare facilities authorize trained staff such as a unit secretary to take off orders if reviewed and signed off by a RN.

Orders for medication contain most but not all the information that must be entered into a MAR. Physicians typically don't specify the exact time to administer scheduled medication. Instead physicians use medical abbreviations to indicate the number of doses to administer to the patient.

The primary nurse is responsible for translating this into a medication schedule when taking off the order using the healthcare facility's policy as a guide. Some healthcare facilities require that medication ordered once a day be given at 10 a.m.

HOW TO TAKE OFF AN ORDER

Let's say that the physician wrote the following prescription:

Lasix 40 mg PO every day

Kcl 20 meq PO every day

These medications above are considered scheduled meds as they indicate that the patient will take these meds every day until the order expiration date—generally 7 days after the initial order is written.

In most systems, the healthcare provider writes the order, and flags the chart. This alerts the unit secretary that there is a new order written for the patient. In a computerized system, the unit secretary enters the order into the chart, leaving it as an unverified order.

The primary RN verifies the order for its accuracy in the computer. This verification is then seen by the pharmacist who will also verify the order, mark it as a verified order, fill it, and send the medication to the unit for the patient.

In a paper system, the same steps would be taken, and the verification by the RN is noted with his or her initials. A copy is sent to pharmacy and the pharmacist will verify the order, fill it, and send it back to the unit.

The nurse then takes off the order by writing it in the MAR as shown in Figure 1.7.

A single order is just that. The nurse can follow that order only once and the order expires. In a computer system, the nurse will enter the order, administer the medication, and chart it as given. The unit secretary can also enter this order and then the system as above will follow for RN/pharmacist verification. In a paper system, the medication is written in the designated area for one-time-only medications and the system above is followed. This is illustrated in Figure 1.8.

PRN is another type of prescription that the physician might write such as:

Zofran 4 mg IV q6h for nausea

Acetaminophen 650 mg PO q6h PRN for temp > 100.5

Medication Administration Record										
Order Date Initials	Exp. Date Time	Medication - Dosage - Frequency Rt. Of Adm.	HR	4/1	4/2	4/3	4/4	4/5	4/6	4/7
4/1 BM	4/7	Lasix 40 mg PO qd	1000							
4/1 BM	4/7	**Kcl 20 meq qd**	1000							

Figure 1.7   Orders are transferred to the MAR.

Code		
O = Omitted	/ = Outdated	Cut = Discontinued
1 = Upper Outer Quadrant R Buttock	7 = Rt. Lateral Thigh	13 = Lt. Anterior Lateral Abdomen
2 = Upper Outer Quadrant L Buttock	8 = Lt. Lateral Thigh	14 = Rt. Posterior Lateral Abdomen
3 = Rt. Deltoid	9 = Rt. Ventroguteal Area	15 = Lt. Posterior Lateral Abdomen
4 = Lt. Deltoid	10 = Lt. Ventrogluteal Area	16 = Rt. Upper Outer Arm
5 = Rt. Mid Anterior Thigh	11 = Abdomen	17 = Lt. Upper Outer Arm
6 = Lt. Mid Anterior Thigh	12 = Rt. Anterior Lateral Abdomen	

Single Orders - Pre-Operatives Stat-Meds						
Order Date Initials	Medication - Dosage - Route	Date Time	Adm. Time	Time Given	Site	Nurse Initial
4/1 BM	MS 2 mg IVP now one time	4/1 1500		1515	IV	BM

Figure 1.8   Write nonschedule medication in the "Single Order" section of the MAR.

Order Date Initials	Stop Date	Medication - Dosage - Frequency Rt. Of Adm.	PRN Medications						
			PRN Medication s- Doses Given						
4/1	4/7	Zofran 4 mg IVP PRN for nausea	Date	4/1					
			Time	08:00					
BM			Init.	BM					
			Site	IV					
4/1	4/7	Acetaminophen 650 mg PO q6h PRN for temp > 100.5	Date	4/1					
			Time	1015					
BM			Init.	BM					
			Site	IV					
			Date						
			Time						
			Init.						
			Site						

Figure 1.9   Medication that can be administered as needed are written in the PRN section.

The system in place for taking off a PRN order would be the same as the system used for a one-time order and/or a scheduled medication. PRN orders are placed in the PRN area of the MAR as shown in Figure 1.9.

Avoid Common Errors When Using the MAR

Errors can occur when taking off orders and recording when medication is administered to a patient resulting in over- or undermedicating the patient or administering incorrect medication.

Steps can be taken to ensure that the most common of these errors are avoided. Here's what you need to do:

- Use abbreviations that are approved by JCAHO and adopted by your healthcare facility. For example, all healthcare facilities require that "daily" replace the abbreviation OD and "every other day" be used in place of QOD. Always write the full word if you are unsure of the abbreviation to write. Refer to your facilities' Dangerous Abbreviations policy for clarification.

- Avoid confusion writing numbers by dropping the zero following a decimal if the dose is a whole number and use a zero to the left of the decimal if the dose is a fraction. This is a JCAHO requirement. Write 1 mg instead of 1.0 mg and 0.5 mg instead of .5 mg.

- Be sure that your full name, title, and initials appear on the MAR before initializing that you administered medication or performed a procedure or diagnostic test.

- Update the MAR immediately after you administer medication to a patient.

- Write legibly on all documents. Assume no one else can read your handwriting so make whatever you can easy to read.

- Write in the MAR the reason for administering PRN medication.

- Note the assessment results on the MAR if particular assessments must be made before administering medication (i.e., the patient's blood pressure before administering blood pressure medication).

HINT If the patient refuses medication, write the patient's own words in quotations in the MAR and/or in the Nurse Progress Notes and other documents required by your healthcare facility.

Documenting Time

Ten o'clock meds are given at what time? This sounds like a joke, but it points to a real problem that occurs in healthcare facilities. There are two 10 o'clocks in a day—morning and evening.

There are two ways in which the time of the day can be specified:

- Use the a.m. (ante meridiem) and p.m. (post meridiem)

- Use **military time**

Many healthcare facilities use military time to avoid any misinterpretation of the time. Military time uses a 24-hour clock that begins with 0000 and ends with 2400. The first hour of the day is 0100, which is 1 a.m. Noon time is 1200. Instead of starting over with 1 p.m., you continue with the sequence. 1 p.m. is 1300. Midnight is 2400.

CONVERTING FROM TRADITIONAL TIME TO MILITARY TIME

Military time is confusing because the first 12 hours of the day is basically the same as using a.m.; however, military time becomes tricky after noon because different numbers are used to indicate the time.

You could count by adding 1 to 12 (noon time) or use these conversion tips.

In the a.m.

1. Remove the colon between hours and minutes.
2. Insert a leading zero if the number is less than 10.

In the p.m.

1. Remove the colon between hours and minutes.
2. Add 1200 to the time.

For example, converting 9:30 a.m. to military time,

a) 930
b) 0930

Converting 2:30 p.m. to military time,

a) 230
b) 230 + 1200 = 1430

CONVERTING MILITARY TIME TO TRADITIONAL TIME

Determine traditional time from military time is straightforward. Here's what you need to do:

If the military time is greater than 1200

1. Subtract 1200 from the time.
2. Insert the colon between the hours and minutes.
3. Insert p.m. at the end of the time.

If the military time is less than 1300

1. Drop the leading zero, if there is one.
2. Insert the colon between the hours and minutes.
3. Insert a.m. at the end of the time.

For example, converting 1430

a) 1430 − 1200 = 230
b) 2:30 p.m.

For example, converting 0930

a) 930

b) 9:30

c) 9:30 a.m.

Medication Labels

The nurse is responsible to make sure that the label on the medication matches the medication in the medication order. If there is a mismatch, the nurse must not administer the medication. The pharmacy is contacted to resolve the conflict.

Some healthcare facilities have a policy that permits the pharmacy to substitute a generic medication for a brand name medication in consultation with the physician without requiring the physician to change the medication order.

STRENGTH OF THE MEDICATION

The medication label specifies the strength of the medication per unit of measure. This is the value that you use to calculate the dose of the medication to administer to the patient.

For example,

- A solution's strength of 30 mg/mL means each milliliter contains 30 milligrams of the medication.

- A tablet's strength of 2 mg per tablet means each tablet contains 2 milligrams of the medication.

- A capsule strength of 10 mg/capsule means each capsule contains 10 milligrams of the medication.

Don't assume that the container holds one dose. Although many healthcare facilities use single-dose containers, you must realize that not all medications come in single-dose containers.

Don't assume that the unit of strength in the medication order is the same as the unit of strength on the medication label. For example, the physician may specify micrograms (mcg) in the medication order and the medication label shows a strength in milligrams (mg). You'll learn how to convert these units in the next chapter.

EXPIRATION DATE

Every medication container specifies an expiration date. Always read the expiration before preparing the medication. Although the pharmacy takes every precaution to purge expired medication, outdated medication can find its way to the nursing unit.

All expired medication should be disposed of immediately according to the healthcare facility's policies.

Summary

A medication order is a prescription a physician writes as part of the patient's treatment plan. The nurse transcribes a medication order to the Medication Administration Record, which is a schedule of the patient's medications and is used to document when and by whom the medication is administered

There are seven parts of a medication order. If any part is missing, the medication order is incomplete and the medication cannot be administered to the patient. The medication order must specify the patient, name of the medication, dose, route, time and frequency, and the physician's signature.

Healthcare facilities have policies that determine when a medication order automatically expires. The nurse must compare the date that the medication order was issued with the healthcare facility's medication order renewal policy before administering medication to the patient.

The nurse must be sure that the medication label matches the medication order. Both the name and strength of the medication on the label must be the same as what the physician ordered otherwise the medication should not be given to the patient. Furthermore, the nurse must be sure that the medication has not expired.

Quiz

1. A nurse who is new to the unit is given a verbal STAT order for medication right before the physician left the unit. The nurse is unsure of the name of the medication. What is the best action to take?

   a. Ask one of the regular nurses what drug the physician normally orders for the patient.

   b. Call the physician.

c. Review the patient's chart to see if the drug might have been previously ordered.

   d. Ask the nurse manager what drug the physician normally orders for the patient.

2. The physician wrote and signed and dated the following order. What would you do?

Mark Jones Patient ID 123345, Room 1220-1, Procardia XL 30 mg p.o.

   a. Calculate the dose and administer the medication.

   b. Administer the medication.

   c. Call the physician.

   d. None of the above.

3. The physician wrote and signed and dated the following order. What would you do?

Mark Jones Patient ID 123345, Room 1220-1, Capoten 12.5 mg p.o. b.i.d.

   a. Calculate the dose and administer the medication.

   b. Administer the medication.

   c. Call the physician.

   d. None of the above.

4. All medication orders are transcribed to the MAR by the physician.

   a. True

   b. False

5. A PRN medication order should

   a. Specify the date and time when the medication is to be given.

   b. Have the nurse manager cosigns the medication order.

   c. Provide instructions to the nurse for when to give the medication.

   d. Be written in front of the patient.

6. Documenting in the MAR that the medication was administered according to the medication order is done

   a. At be beginning of the shift

   b. Immediately after the medication is administered

   c. At the end of the shift

   d. When the nurse has a free moment

7. An example of taking off orders is the process of

   a. Transcribing a medication order to the MAR

   b. Comparing the medication to the MAR

   c. Comparing the medication to the medication order

   d. Receiving an update about a patient at the beginning of the shift

8. A medication order is written as q6h requiring the patient to receive the medication every 6 hours. Who determines the exact hour to give the medication?

   a. The healthcare facility's policy

   b. The patient

   c. The nurse manager

   d. The physician

9. What is the best action to take when a medication order is illegible?

   a. Call the physician

   b. Ask another nurse to help read the medication order

   c. Look up the medication in the drug book

   d. Look up the medication in the chart

10. How is 10 a.m. written in military time?

    a. 01000

    b. 010:00

    c. 10

    d. 010

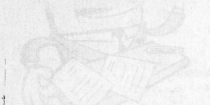

CHAPTER 2

CHAPTER 2

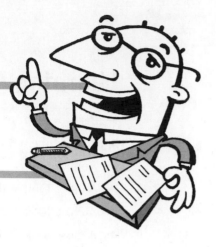

The Formula Method

Based on the medical diagnosis, the physician prescribes a dose of the medication that will improve the patient's condition. Sometimes this is the same dose that appears on the medication label, which means that the patient receives the complete content of the container.

However, the medication might be a different dose and thus requires the nurse to calculate the amount of medication to administer to the patient.

Two methods are used to calculate the dose: the formula method and the proportion method. Both methods arrive at the same dose. Whatever method you choose, it is best to stick with it for all dose calculations to avoid errors.

In this chapter, you'll learn the formula method of calculating the dose. The proportion method is explained in the next chapter.

Learning Objectives

➤ Parts of the formula

➤ Calculating a dose using the formula method

➤ Rounding tips

➤ A close look at the metric system

➤ A close look at the apothecaries system

➤ A close look at the household system

Key Words

Apothecaries system	Meter
Dose on hand	Metric system
Dose ordered	Milligram (mg)
Dram	Milliliter (mL)
Grain (gr)	Minim
Gram	Ounce
Household system	Prefix
International System of Units (SI)	Quantity
Liter	The formula method

Parts of the Formula

The **formula method** has been adopted by many nurses because the formula is straightforward and easy to understand and use. If you can divide and multiply, then you won't have any trouble using the formula method.

There are three parts to the formula:

• **Dose ordered:** The dose ordered is the dose specified in the medication order.

• **Dose on hand:** The dose on hand is the dose specified on the medication label (Figure 2.1)

• **Quantity:** The quantity is the unit of measure on the medication label that contains the dose. (Figure 2.1)

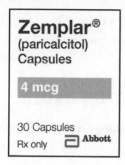

Figure 2.1   The dose on hand for ZEMPLAR is
4 mcg and the quantity is 1 capsule.

WRITING THE FORMULA

The secret to using the formula to calculate the dose is to properly set up the equation. The equation is written as:

$$\frac{\text{Ordered}}{\text{On hand}} \times \text{quantity} = \text{dose}$$

Some nurses use a shorter way to write this formula:

$$\frac{O}{H} \times Q = D$$

Calculating a Dose Using the Formula Method

There are a few steps to follow to calculate the dose using the formula method. However, avoid the trap. Be careful when performing these steps. Because these steps are simple, there is a tendency to rush through the calculations, which results in errors. Remember that an error means that you'll be giving your patient the wrong dose.

Here are the steps:

1. Read the medication order and identify the information you need for the formula.

2. Read the medication label and identify the information you need for the formula.

3. Insert the values from the medication order and medication label into the formula.

4. Calculate.

5. Repeat steps 1 through 4 to check your answer.

READING THE MEDICATION ORDER

The physician wrote the following order for Dilantin for your patient. Your job is to calculate the number of milliliters of Dilantin to give to your patient.

Dilantin 100 mg p.o. t.i.d.

What information in this order do you need to calculate the dose for your patient? Let's take apart this order.

- The name of the medication is Dilantin.

- The dose ordered is 100 milligrams.

- The medication is P.O. which means it is given by mouth.

- The medication is given t.i.d., which means it is given three times a day.

Only the dose ordered is needed for the calculation. Although the name of the medication must match the medication label, the name isn't used in the calculation. Likewise, you don't need to know how to administer the medication and the number of times to administer to calculate the dose.

READING THE MEDICATION LABEL

The pharmacy delivered Dilantin to the unit. The following is a portion of the information contained on the label.

Dilantin suspension 125 mg/5 mL

What information on this order do you need to calculate the dose for your patient? Let's take apart this label.

- The name of the medication is Dilantin.

- The dose is 125 milligrams in 5 milliliters.

The information needed for the formula is the dose on hand, which is 125 mg, and the quantity, which is 5 mL. The name of the medication isn't required by the formula.

HINT *Besides the dose, the medication label also contains the total quantity of medication in the container. Don't confuse the dose volume with the quantity in the container. In a single dose container called a unit dose, the quantity of the medication in the container is the same as in the dose. In a multiple dose container, the quantity is larger than the dose.*

INSERTING VALUES INTO THE FORMULA

Let's insert values from the medication order and the medication label into the dose calculation formula. When doing so, it is very important that you include both the value and the unit of measurement (i.e., mg, mL).

As you'll learn later in this chapter, the unit of measurement specified in the medication order may differ from the unit measurement on the medication label. You cannot calculate unlike unit of measurements, therefore you'll need to convert to the same unit of measurement. You'll see how this is done later in this chapter.

For now, remember to specify the unit of measurement in the formula. This will alert you if you need to convert units. In this example, the same units of measurements are used so there is no conversion.

$$\frac{100 \text{ mg}}{125 \text{ mg}} \times 5 \text{ mL} = D$$

CALCULATING THE FORMULA

There are two mathematical operations that must be performed to calculate the dose. These are division and multiplication.

1. First divide the dose on hand into the dose ordered.

$$\frac{100 \text{ mg}}{125 \text{ mg}} = 0.8$$

2. Next, multiply by 5 mL to calculate the dose to administer to the patient.

$$0.8 \times 5 \text{ mL} = 4 \text{ mL}$$

You will administer 4 mL of Dilantin to the patient.

Rounding Tips

In the real world and on dose calculation exams, calculated values are not always in round numbers. You will have decimal places in your calculation. Here's how you need to manage decimal places.

- Round only the final value that you calculate and leave the intermediate values unrounded. If you don't, then you answer might be incorrect although you had the values in the proper position in the formula and your math was correct.
- Round two decimal places only.
- Round only the third decimal place.
- Round up when the third decimal place is five or greater.
- Round down when the third decimal place is less than five.

Practice Drill 2.1—the Formula Method

Practicing is the best way to learn how to calculate a dose. Here is a drill of practical problems that you might find when you are caring for patients in a healthcare facility. Follow the steps discussed previously in this chapter and calculate the correct dose for your patients.

1. Medication order: Capoten 6.25 mg P.O. q8h
   Medication label: Capoten 12.5 mg per tablet

   How many tablets to administer to the patient?

2. Medication order: Morphine sulfate 2 mg I.M. STAT
   Medication label: Morphine sulfate 10 mg/mL

   How many milliliters to administer to the patient?

3. Medication order: Xanax 0.25 mg P.O. daily
   Medication label: Xanax 0.5 mg per tablet

   How many tablets to administer to the patient?

4. Medication order: Charcotabs 520 mg P.O. STAT
   Medication label: Charcotabs 260 mg per tablet

   How many tablets to administer to the patient?

5. Medication order: Demerol 75 mg I.M. PRN
   Medication label: Demerol 50 mg/mL

   How many milliliters to administer to the patient?

6. Medication order: Allopurinol 300 mg P.O. daily
   Medication label: Allopurinol 100 mg per tablet

   How many tablets to administer to the patient?

7. Medication order: Garamycin 60 mg I.M. STAT
   Medication label: Garamycin 80 mg/mL

   How many milliliters to administer to the patient?

8. Medication order: Corophyllin 500 mg q6h
   Medication label: Corophyllin 250 mg/1 rectal suppository

   How many tablets to administer to the patient?

9. Medication order: Colace 50 mg P.O. daily
   Medication label: Colace 100 mg/capsule

   How many capsules to administer to the patient?

10. Medication order: Azulfidine 1000 mg P.O. daily
    Medication label: Azulfidine 500 mg per tablet

    How many tablets to administer to the patient?

Solutions to Practice Drill 2.1—the Formula Method

1. $\dfrac{6.25 \text{ mg}}{12.5 \text{ mg}} \times 1 \text{ tablet} = 0.5 \text{ tablet}$

2. $\dfrac{2 \text{ mg}}{10 \text{ mg}} \times 1 \text{ mL} = 0.2 \text{ mL}$

3. $\dfrac{0.25 \text{ mg}}{0.5 \text{ mg}} \times 1 \text{ tablet} = 0.5 \text{ tablet}$

4. $\dfrac{520 \text{ mg}}{260 \text{ mg}} \times 1 \text{ tablet} = 2 \text{ tablets}$

5. $\dfrac{75 \text{ mg}}{50 \text{ mg}} \times 1 \text{ mL} = 1.5 \text{ mL}$

6. $\dfrac{300 \text{ mg}}{100 \text{ mg}} \times 1 \text{ tablet} = 3 \text{ tablets}$

7. $\dfrac{60 \text{ mg}}{80 \text{ mg}} \times 1 \text{ mL} = 0.75 \text{ mL}$

8. $\dfrac{500 \text{ mg}}{250 \text{ mg}} \times 1 \text{ rectal suppository} = 2 \text{ rectal suppositories}$

9. $\dfrac{50 \text{ mg}}{100 \text{ mg}} \times 1 \text{ capsule} = 0.5 \text{ capsule}$

10. $\dfrac{1000 \text{ mg}}{500 \text{ mg}} \times 1 \text{ tablet} = 2 \text{ tablets}$

A Close Look at the Metric System

Medication is specified using the **metric system**, which is also referred to as the **International System of Units (SI)**. There are three basic units of measurement in the metric system. These are:

- **Gram:** A gram is used to measure weight.
- **Liter:** A liter is used to measure a volume.
- **Meter:** A meter is used to measure length.

Weight and volume are used in dose calculations. Length is not used to calculate a dose; however, it is used to measure a patient's height.

A **prefix** is used to identify the numeric value of the unit. That is, the number of grams, liters, and meters. Table 2.1 shows the prefixes that are commonly used in medication.

For example, a milliliter is one thousandths of a liter and a milligram is one thousandths of a gram. Table 2.2 contains abbreviations for metric units commonly used in dose calculations.

Table 2.1 Prefixes Used for Medication

Prefix	Numeric value
Kilo	One thousand times (1000)
Centi	One hundredths of (0.01)
Milli	One thousandths of (0.001)
Micro	One millionth of (0.000001)

Table 2.2   Abbreviations of Units

Abbreviation	Unit
g	gram
mg	milligram
mcg	microgram
L	liter
mL	milliliter
kg	kilogram

HINT *Don't memorize the numeric value of a prefix. Instead, focus on the relative size such as milli is larger than a micro. This helps with your critical thinking skills to determine if something is large or small.*

CONVERTING METRIC UNITS

There will be times when the unit in the medication order will be different from the unit used on the medication label. For example, the physician might specify micrograms (mcg) and the label reads milligrams (mg).

This doesn't mean that the physician made an error or that there is a misprint on the medication label. It simply means that you must convert values to the same unit of measure before calculating the dose.

The conversion process is straightforward because you convert using a factor of 1000 and by moving the decimal point either three places to the left or right.

Let's see how this works. Say that the order is for 50 mg and the medication on hand is in micrograms. You must convert the 50 mg into micrograms before calculating the dose.

1. The first step is to determine if you are converting from a larger to a smaller amount or from a smaller to a larger amount. In this example, 50 mg is being converted to micrograms. Therefore, a larger amount (milligrams) is being converted to a smaller amount.

2. The next step is to set up the conversion equation.

   50 mg = ? mcg

3. Multiply by 1000 when converting a large value to a small value. Divide by 1000 when converting a small value to a large value. In this example, you multiply 50 mg by 1000 to convert to micrograms.

   50 mg = 50,000 mcg

HINT *Memorize:*

- *When converting larger to smaller, move the decimal point three places to the right.*
- *When converting smaller to large, move the decimal point three places to the left.*

Always place a zero to the left of the decimal point if there isn't a whole number. This makes it easy to read the decimal point and avoids errors.

A Close Look at the Apothecaries System

The **apothecaries system** is an older system for measuring weight and volume and has been widely replaced by the metric system; although some physicians might prescribe medications using the apothecaries units. Values measured in the apothecaries system are approximations and not exact as in the metric system.

Weights are measured using grain.

- **Grain:** A grain is abbreviated as gr.

Volume is measured in three units

- **Minim:** A minim is abbreviated as m. Healthcare facilities also discourage using minims.
- **Dram:** A dram is a unit used to measure dry medication. It is abbreviated as dr. Although you'll find drams on medication cup, the use of this measure has been discouraged by healthcare facilities.
- **Ounce:** An ounce is abbreviated as oz and is also used in the **household system** of measurement.

HINT *Focus on learning to convert a grain to a gram and a milligram to a grain. Although you might not have to convert these units in the healthcare facility, you may have to convert them on a test. Also to remember is that the unit of measurement precedes the value when using grain. Here are the conversion factors to memorize.*

gr 15 = 1 g
60 mg = gr 1

A Close Look at the Household System

The household system is a system of measurement used primarily for cooking and is used by patients to measure medication at home because home utensils are gauged for the household system. You'll need to convert the medication order dose from metric to household system.

The household system measures volume using the units shown in Table 2.3.

Two medications that you'll frequently need to convert to the household systems are Maalox and GoLytely. Maalox is used as an antacid and a laxative depending on the dose prescribed by the physician. GoLytely is a bowel preparation that is prescribed prior to a colonoscopy. Both are usually taken by the patient at home.

Let's say that the physician wrote a medication order for Maalox 30 mL. The patient probably doesn't have a metric utensil at home to measure this amount of Maalox. Therefore, the dose must be converted to a unit of the household system.

There are three choices:

- Two tablespoons
- Six teaspoons
- One cup

The dose for GoLytely is typically 1.2 L. The patient has a cup (8 oz) at home. You must calculate the number of cups of GoLytely that the patient must take. Looking at Table 2.4, you'll notice that there isn't a simple factor to use to convert liters to a cup. Therefore, you'll need to perform intermediate conversions.

Here's how to perform this conversion.

1. Convert 1.2 L into milliliters. You're going from large to small so move the decimal point three positions to the right.

   1.2 L = 1200 mL

Table 2.3   Abbreviations of Units

Abbreviation	Unit
oz	ounce
tbs or T	tablespoon
tsp or t	teaspoon
cup	cup
pt	pint
qt	quart
gal	gallon

Table 2.4 Conversion Factors from Metric
to the Household System

1 oz = 30 mL
1 tbs = 15 mL
1 tsp = 5 mL
1 cup = 240 mL = 8 oz
1 pt = 500 mL = 32 oz
1 qt = 1000 mL = 32 oz
1 gal = 4 qt

2. Convert 1200 mL to cups. Table 2.4 states that 240 mL equals 1 cup. Therefore, dividing 1200 mL by 240 mL will result in the number of cups GoLytely the patient needs to take.

$$\frac{1200 \text{ mL}}{240 \text{ mL}} = 5 \text{ cups}$$

Practice Drill 2.2—Converting Values

Here is a drill of practical problems that you'll need to convert units first and then calculate the dose. Calculate the dose by following steps discussed previously in this chapter.

1. Medication order: Vitamin B12 1 mg P.O. daily
   Medication label: Vitamin 500 mcg per tablet

   How many tablets to administer to the patient?

2. Medication order: Erythromycin 100 mg I.V.
   Medication label: Erythromycin 1g/30 mL

   How many milliliters to administer to the patient?

3. Medication order: Methozamine HCl 0.015 g I.M. daily
   Medication label: Methozamine HCl 10 mg/mL

   How many milliliters to administer to the patient?

4. Medication order: Quinidine Sulfate 400 mg P.O. daily
   Medication Label: Quinidine Sulfate 0.2 g per tablet

   How many tablets to administer to the patient?

5. Medication order: Lopid 0.6 g P.O. daily
   Medication label: Lopid 600 mg per tablet
   How many tablets to administer to the patient?

6. Medication order: Amphojet 5 mL P.O. daily

   The patient has a teaspoon available at home.

   How many teaspoons should the patient take of Amphojet?

7. Medication order: Maalox 1 oz P.O. daily
   The patient has a tablespoon available at home.

   How many tablespoons should the patient take of Maalox?

8. Medication order: Water 1 gal P.O. daily
   The patient has an 8 oz cup available at home.

   How many cups should the patient take of water?

9. Medication order: Milk of Magnesia 30 mL P.O. daily
   The patient has a tablespoon available at home.

   How many tablespoons should the patient take of Milk of Magnesia?

10. Medication order: fruit juice 4000 mL P.O. daily
    The patient has 1 qt container available at home.

    How many quarts should the patient take of fruit juice?

Solutions to Practice Drill 2.2—Converting Values

1. Convert milligrams (mg) to micrograms (mcg) because the medication on hand is in micrograms.

   $1 \text{ mg} \times 1000 = 1000 \text{ mcg}$

   Calculate the dose

   $$\frac{1000 \text{ mg}}{500 \text{ mcg}} \times 1 \text{ tablet} = 2 \text{ tablets}$$

2. Convert milligrams (mg) to grams (g) because the medication on hand is in grams.

   $$\frac{100 \text{ mg}}{1000} = 0.1 \text{ g}$$

   Calculate the dose

   $$\frac{0.1 \text{ g}}{1 \text{ g}} \times 30 \text{ mL} = 3 \text{ mL}$$

3. Convert grams (g) to milligrams (mg) because the medication is in milligrams.

   $0.015 \text{ g} \times 1000 = 15 \text{ mg}$

Calculate the dose

$$\frac{15 \text{ mg}}{10 \text{ mg}} \times 1 \text{ mL} = 1.5 \text{ mL}$$

4. Convert milligrams (mg) to grams (g) because the medication on hand is in grams.

$$\frac{400 \text{ mg}}{1000} = 0.4 \text{ g}$$

Calculate the dose

$$\frac{0.4 \text{ g}}{0.2 \text{ g}} \times 1 \text{ tablet} = 2 \text{ tablets}$$

5. Convert grams (g) to milligrams (mg) because the medication is in milligrams

$$0.6 \text{ g} \times 1000 = 600 \text{ mg}$$

Calculate the dose

$$\frac{600 \text{ mg}}{600 \text{ mg}} \times 1 \text{ tablet} = 1 \text{ tablet}$$

6. 5 mL = 1 teaspoon

7. a) 1 oz = 30 mL

 b) 1 tablespoon = 15 mL

 c) $\dfrac{30 \text{ mL}}{15 \text{ mL}} = 2 \text{ tablespoons}$

8. a) 1 gal = 4 qt

 b) 1 qt = 32 oz

 c) 4 qt × 32 oz = 128 oz = 1 gal

 d) $\dfrac{128 \text{ oz}}{8 \text{ oz}} = 16 \text{ cups}$

9. a) 1 tablespoon = 15 mL

 b) $\dfrac{30 \text{ mL}}{15 \text{ mL}} = 2 \text{ tablespoons}$

10. a) 1 qt = 1000 mL

 b) $\dfrac{4000 \text{ mL}}{1000 \text{ mL}} = 4 \text{ qt}$

Summary

The formula method is one of the two methods used to calculate the dose to administer to a patient. The other is the proportion method. Stay with one method to avoid the risk of errors in your calculations.

In the formula method, the dose ordered is divided by the dose on hand and then multiplied by the quantity. Both the dose ordered and dose on hand must be in the same unit of measure. If not, then convert the dose ordered to the units of the dose on hand before calculating.

Most medication use the metric system known as the International System of Units (SI) where the prefix of the unit describes its relative size. Move the decimal point three places to the right when converting a small unit to a larger unit. Move the decimal point three places to the left when converting a large unit to a small unit. This depends on what the physician ordered.

The apothecaries system is another system of measurement that is discouraged by healthcare facilities and therefore is rarely used today. The household system of measurement is used by patients at home to measure medication. You'll need to convert the dose in the metric system to the household system whenever the patient is going to self medicate using cups, teaspoons, and other utensils found around the house.

When calculating, round only after all the calculations are completed. Don't round intermediate values. Calculate to three decimal places and round to two decimal places. Round up when the value is 5 or greater and round down if the value is less than 5.

Quiz

1. The medication order is for Lanoxin 0.50 mg and the pharmacy delivered Lanoxin 0.25 mg per tablet. What dose would you administer to the patient?

    a. 2 tablets

    b. A half of a table

    c. 1 tablet

    d. 2.5 tablets

2. The medication order is for Motrin 0.6 g and the pharmacy delivered Motrin 400 mg per tablet. What dose would you administer to the patient?

    a. 1 tablet

    b. 1.25 tablets

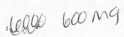

c.   1.5 tablets

    d.   0.5 tablets

3. The medication order is for Decadron 3 mg and the pharmacy delivered Decadron 0.75 mg per tablet. What dose would you administer to the patient?

    a.   2.5 tablets

    b.   2 tablets

    c.   4 tablets

    d.   4.5 tablets

4. The medication order is for Milk of Magnesia 5 mL. You should tell the patient to use 1 teaspoon of Milk of Magnesia.

    a.   True

    b.   False

5. The medication order is for Norpace 0.30 g and the pharmacy delivered Norpace 150 mg per tablet. What dose would you administer to the patient?

    a.   2.5 tablets   300 mg

    b.   2 tablets

    c.   3 tablets

    d.   3.5 tablets

6. The medication order is for Vistaril 25 mg and the pharmacy delivered Vistaril 50 mg/mL. What dose would you administer to the patient?

    a.   2.5 mL

    b.   2 mL

    c.   1 mL

    d.   0.5 mL

7. The medication order is for Ampicillin 1 g and the pharmacy delivered Ampicillin 500 mg per capsule. What dose would you administer to the patient?

    a.   2.5 capsules

    b.   2 capsules

    c.   3 capsules

    d.   3.5 capsules

8. The medication order is for Dilantin 50 mg and the pharmacy delivered Dilantin 125 mg/5 mL. What dose would you administer to the patient?

   a. 2 mL

   b. 2.5 mL

   c. 3 mL

   d. 4.5 mL

$$\frac{125\,mg}{5\,mL} \times \frac{50\,mg}{X}$$

$$\frac{250}{125} = \frac{125\,X}{125}$$

9. The medication order is for Synthroid 0.05 mg and the pharmacy delivered Synthroid 25 mcg per tablet. What dose would you administer to the patient?

   a. 2 tablets   50 mcg

   b. 2.5 tablets

   c. 3 tablets

   d. 3.5 tablets

10. The medication order is for Demerol 50 mg and the pharmacy delivered Demerol 75 mg per mL. What dose would you administer to the patient?

   a. 0.60 mL

   b. 0.66 mL

   c. 0.67 mL

   d. 0.70 mL

$$\frac{75\,mg}{1\,mL} \times \frac{50\,mg}{X}$$

$$\frac{50}{75} = \frac{75\,X}{75}$$

$$75\overline{)50.0} \quad 0.666\,\text{uu}$$
$$\underline{-450}$$
$$500$$

CHAPTER 3

The Ratio-Proportion Method

Ratio-proportion is another method used for calculating the dose to administer to patient. It is similar to the formula method that you learned in the previous chapter. Both methods arrive at the same dose. Only the calculation is different.

The goal of the ratio-proportion method is to solve for X using a simple algebraic expression. X is the dose. Other elements of the expression are given in the medication order and on the medication label.

You'll learn how to use the ratio-proportion method in this chapter and be in the position to choose the ratio-proportion method or the formula method to calculate the dose of medication for your patients.

Learning Objectives

➤ Understanding the ratio

➤ The ratio-proportion expression

Key Words

Known value

Proportion

Ratio

Unknown value

Understanding the Ratio

Before diving into math, step back a moment and take another look at the dose on a medication label.

25 mg/mL

This is saying that every milliliter of fluid contains 25 mg of medication. In other words if you draw up 1 mL from the container into a syringe, the syringe will have 25 mg of medication.

Suppose you drew up 2 mL into the syringe. How many milligrams of medication are in the syringe? You probably answered this in your head because intuitively you realize if the quantity (mL) doubled so must the amount of medication (mg). There are 50 mg of medication in the syringe.

Intuitively you used ratio-proportion to calculate the dose.

PROPORTION

Proportion means there is a linear relationship between two values. This simply means that an increase in one value causes the other value to increase at the same rate. This relationship between the dose and quantity is printed on the medication label.

The pharmaceutical that made the medication determined the proportion through research and clinical trials that occur before the Food and Drug Administration approved the medication for clinical use.

RATIO

A **ratio** is a way to write the proportional relationship of two values. There are two ways that you'll see a ratio written. The first is the way the ratio appears on the medication label such as

$$25 \text{ mg/mL}$$

The other way is to write the ratio in an expression using the colon instead of the forward slash such as

$$25 \text{ mg} : \text{mL}$$

Both of these are saying the same thing, that is, there are 25 mg in each milliliter of fluid in the container.

The Ratio-Proportion Expression

The ratio-proportion expression is divided into two components: known and unknown. The known component is the ratio on the medication label. The unknown component is the medication order. As you'll recall from the last chapter, the medication order specifies a dose but not the quantity. You must calculate the quantity.

Let's say that physician ordered 50 mg of a medication. The medication label reads 100 mg/mL. Here's how to represent this in the ratio-proportion expression.

$$100 \text{ mg} : 1 \text{ mL} = 50 \text{ mg} : X \text{ mL}$$

The known (medication label), the left of the equal sign, is a ratio. The unknown (medication order), to the right of the equal sign, is also a ratio except an X is used to represent the quantity. The objective is to solve X.

The proportional relationship between the dose and the quantity of the medication label is the key to calculating the dose. You apply this proportion to the unknown side of the ratio-proportion expression to determine the dose to administer to the patient.

Calculating Using the Ratio-Proportional Expression

The initial step in calculating the ratio-proportional expression is to transform the ratio-proportional expression into two fractions by replacing the colon with a division sign as shown here:

$$\frac{100 \text{ mg}}{1 \text{ mL}} = \frac{50 \text{ mg}}{X \text{ mL}}$$

The next step is to cross multiply. When cross multiplying, apply the rules of algebra and move values from the left side of the expression to the right side so that X is on the left side of the expression. When a value is moved, its operation is reversed.

Move 100 mg to the right side and X mL to the left side as shown here:

$$\frac{X \text{ mL}}{1 \text{ mL}} = \frac{50 \text{ mg}}{100 \text{ mg}}$$

Next move 1 mL to the right side of the expression. The operation on the left side of the expression is division, therefore the operation is reversed to multiplication when the 1 mL quantity is moved to the right side of the expression as shown here:

$$X \text{ mL} = \frac{50 \text{ mg}}{100 \text{ mg}} \times 1 \text{ mL}$$

The last step is to calculate the expression.

$$X \text{ mL} = 0.5 \times 1 \text{ mL}$$
$$X \text{ mL} = 0.5 \text{ mL}$$

HINTS *Here are few suggestions to remember when using ratio-proportion method to calculate the dose to administer to your patient.*

- The known (medication label) ratio is on the left of the equal sign and the unknown (medication order) is on the right.
- Set up each ratio the same way—dose: quantity

- Always label each value in each ratio.

- Make sure like units of measurements are used. If the unit of measurement in the medication order is different than the unit of measurement on the medication label, then convert the medication order to the medication label unit of measurement.

- Only round the value of *X*. Don't round intermediate values.

- *X* must be the lone value to the left of the equal sign

Practice Drill 3.1—the Ratio-Proportion Method

Try your hand at calculating the same doses as you calculated in the previous chapter only this time use the ratio-proportion method. Take your time and carefully follow the steps discussed previously in this chapter. Compare the ratio-proportion method to the formula method (Chapter 2) when you finish this drill.

1. Medication order: Capoten 6.25 mg P.O. q8h
   Medication label: Capoten 12.5 mg per tablet

   How many tablets to administer to the patient?

2. Medication order: Morphine sulfate 2 mg I.M. STAT
   Medication label: Morphine sulfate 10 mg/mL

   How many milliliters to administer to the patient?

3. Medication order: Xanax 0.25 mg P.O. daily
   Medication label: Xanax 0.5 mg per tablet

   How many tablets to administer to the patient?

4. Medication order: Charcotabs 520 mg P.O. STAT
   Medication label: Charcotabs 260 mg per tablet

   How many tablets to administer to the patient?

5. Medication order: Demerol 75 mg I.M. PRN
   Medication label: Demerol 50 mg/mL

   How many milliliters to administer to the patient?

6. Medication order: Allopurinol 300 mg P.O. daily
   Medication label: Allopurinol 100 mg per tablet

   How many tablets to administer to the patient?

7. Medication order: Garamycin 60 mg I.M. STAT
   Medication label: Garamycin 80 mg/mL

   How many milliliters to administer to the patient?

8. Medication order: Corophyllin 500 mg q6h PRN
   Medication label: Corophyllin 250 mg/1 rectal suppository

   How many tablets to administer to the patient?

9. Medication order: Colace 50 mg P.O. daily
   Medication label: Colace 100 mg/capsule

   How many capsules to administer to the patient?

10. Medication order: Azulfidine 1000 mg P.O. daily
    Medication label: Azulfidine 500 mg per tablet

    How many tablets to administer to the patient?

Solutions to Practice Drill 3.1—the Ratio-Proportion Method

1. $$\frac{12.5\ mg}{1\ tablet} = \frac{6.25\ mg}{X\ tablet}$$

   $$\frac{X\ tablet}{1\ tablet} = \frac{6.25\ mg}{12.5\ mg}$$

   $$X\ tablet = \frac{6.25\ mg}{12.5\ mg} \times 1\ tablet$$

   $$X\ tablet = 0.5 \times 1\ tablet$$

   $$X\ tablet = 0.5\ tablet$$

2. $$\frac{10\ mg}{1\ mL} = \frac{2\ mg}{X\ mL}$$

   $$\frac{X\ mL}{1\ mL} = \frac{2\ mg}{10\ mg}$$

   $$X\ mL = \frac{2\ mg}{10\ mg} \times 1\ mL$$

   $$X\ mL = 0.2 \times 1\ mL$$

   $$X\ mL = 0.2\ mL$$

3. $\dfrac{0.5 \text{ mg}}{1 \text{ tablet}} = \dfrac{0.25 \text{ mg}}{X \text{ tablet}}$

$\dfrac{X \text{ tablet}}{1 \text{ tablet}} = \dfrac{0.25 \text{ mg}}{0.5 \text{ mg}}$

$X \text{ tablet} = \dfrac{0.25 \text{ mg}}{0.5 \text{ mg}} \times 1 \text{ tablet}$

$X \text{ tablet} = 0.5 \times 1 \text{ tablet}$

$X \text{ tablet} = 0.5 \text{ tablet}$

4. $\dfrac{260 \text{ mg}}{1 \text{ tablet}} = \dfrac{520 \text{ mg}}{X \text{ tablet}}$

$\dfrac{X \text{ tablet}}{1 \text{ tablet}} = \dfrac{520 \text{ mg}}{260 \text{ mg}}$

$X \text{ tablet} = \dfrac{520 \text{ mg}}{260 \text{ mg}} \times 1 \text{ tablet}$

$X \text{ tablet} = 2 \times 1 \text{ tablet}$

$X \text{ tablet} = 2 \text{ tablets}$

5. $\dfrac{50 \text{ mg}}{1 \text{ mL}} = \dfrac{75 \text{ mg}}{X \text{ mL}}$

$\dfrac{X \text{ mL}}{1 \text{ mL}} = \dfrac{75 \text{ mg}}{50 \text{ mg}}$

$X \text{ mL} = \dfrac{75 \text{ mg}}{50 \text{ mg}} \times 1 \text{ mL}$

$X \text{ mL} = 1.5 \times 1 \text{ mL}$

$X \text{ mL} = 1.5 \text{ mL}$

6. $\dfrac{100 \text{ mg}}{1 \text{ tablet}} = \dfrac{300 \text{ mg}}{X \text{ tablet}}$

$\dfrac{X \text{ tablet}}{1 \text{ tablet}} = \dfrac{300 \text{ mg}}{100 \text{ mg}}$

$X \text{ tablet} = \dfrac{300 \text{ mg}}{100 \text{ mg}} \times 1 \text{ tablet}$

$X \text{ tablet} = 3 \times 1 \text{ tablet}$

$X \text{ tablet} = 3 \text{ tablets}$

7. $$\frac{80 \text{ mg}}{1 \text{ mL}} = \frac{60 \text{ mg}}{X \text{ mL}}$$

$$\frac{X \text{ mL}}{1 \text{ mL}} = \frac{60 \text{ mg}}{80 \text{ mg}}$$

$$X \text{ mL} = \frac{60 \text{ mg}}{80 \text{ mg}} \times 1 \text{ mL}$$

$$X \text{ mL} = 0.75 \times 1 \text{ mL}$$

$$X \text{ mL} = 0.75 \text{ mL}$$

8. $$\frac{250 \text{ mg}}{1 \text{ rectal suppository}} = \frac{500 \text{ mg}}{X \text{ rectal suppository}}$$

$$\frac{X \text{ rectal suppository}}{1 \text{ rectal suppository}} = \frac{500 \text{ mg}}{250 \text{ mg}}$$

$$X \text{ rectal suppository} = \frac{500 \text{ mg}}{250 \text{ mg}} \times 1 \text{ rectal suppository}$$

$$X \text{ rectal suppository} = 2 \times 1 \text{ rectal suppository}$$

$$X \text{ rectal suppository} = 2 \text{ rectal suppositories}$$

9. $$\frac{100 \text{ mg}}{1 \text{ capsule}} = \frac{50 \text{ mg}}{X \text{ capsule}}$$

$$\frac{X \text{ capsule}}{1 \text{ capsule}} = \frac{50 \text{ mg}}{100 \text{ mg}}$$

$$X \text{ capsule} = \frac{50 \text{ mg}}{100 \text{ mg}} \times 1 \text{ capsule}$$

$$X \text{ capsule} = 0.5 \times 1 \text{ capsule}$$

$$X \text{ capsule} = 0.5 \text{ capsule}$$

10. $$\frac{500 \text{ mg}}{1 \text{ tablet}} = \frac{1000 \text{ mg}}{X \text{ tablet}}$$

$$\frac{X \text{ tablet}}{1 \text{ tablet}} = \frac{1000 \text{ mg}}{500 \text{ mg}}$$

$$X \text{ tablet} = \frac{1000 \text{ mg}}{500 \text{ mg}} \times 1 \text{ tablet}$$

$$X \text{ tablet} = 2 \times 1 \text{ tablet}$$

$$X \text{ tablet} = 2 \text{ tablets}$$

Summary

The ratio-proportion method is used to calculate a dose and arrives at the same dose as calculated by the formula method. Two ratios are used: known and unknown.

The known is the ratio of medication and quantity found on the medication label. The unknown is the medication ordered and the quantity that is administered to the patient, which you are calculating.

Both ratios are converted to fractions and the dose is calculated by using cross multiplication. The dose is the same dose that is calculated by using the formula method.

Quiz

1. The medication order is for Guaifenesin 100 mg and the pharmacy delivered Guaifenesin 200 mg/5 mL. What dose would you administer to the patient?

   a.   2 mL

   b.   2.5 mL

   c.   1 mL

   d.   1.5 mL

2. The medication order is for Valproic 1.5 mg and the pharmacy delivered Valproic 3 mg/mL. What dose would you administer to the patient?

   a.   1 mL

   b.   1.25 mL

   c.   1.5 mL

   d.   0.5 mL

3. The medication order is for Xanax 4000 mcg and the pharmacy delivered Xanax 2 mg/tablet. What dose would you administer to the patient?

   a.   2.5 tablets

   b.   2 tablets   *2mg = 2000 mcg*

   c.   4 tablets

   d.   4.5 tablets

4. The medication order is for Dimelor 2.5 mg. The medication label reads Dimelor 5 mg/tablet. You should administer a half of tablet.

a. True

b. False

5. The medication order is for Demerol 75 mg and the pharmacy delivered Demerol 25 mg/0.5 mL. What dose would you administer to the patient?

   a. 1.5 mL

   b. 1 mL

   c. 2 mL

   d. 2.5 mL

6. The medication order is for Chloral Hydrate 50 mg and the pharmacy delivered Chloral Hydrate 25 mg/2 mL. What dose would you administer to the patient?

   a. 3 mL

   b. 3.5 mL

   c. 4 mL

   d. 4.5 mL

7. The medication order is for Norvasc 500 mg and the pharmacy delivered Norvasc 250 mg/tablet. What dose would you administer to the patient?

   a. 2.5 capsules

   b. 2 capsules

   c. 3 capsules

   d. 3.5 capsules

8. The medication order is for Keflex 250 mg and the pharmacy delivered Keflex 125 mg/capsule. What dose would you administer to the patient?

   a. 1 capsule

   b. 1.5 capsules

   c. 2 capsules

   d. 2.5 capsules

9. The medication order is for Allopurinol 105 mg and the pharmacy delivered Allopurinol 30 mg/tablet. What dose would you administer to the patient?

   a. 2 tablets

   b. 2.5 tablets

   c. 3 tablets

   d. 3.5 tablets

10. The medication order is for Azulfidine 250 mg and the pharmacy delivered Azulfidine 50 mg/tablet. What dose would you administer to the patient?

   a.   4 tablets

   b.   4.5 tablets

   c.   5 tablets

   d.   5.5 tablets

CHAPTER 4

Intravenous Calculations

Your patient may require intravenous (I.V.) therapy, which is a continuous flow of medication delivered into the patient's vein over a period of time. How much medication the patient receives depends on the rate of flow of the I.V.

The rate is controlled by setting the number of drops of fluid that are administered to the patient each minute. Alternatively, the rate is controlled by the number of milliliters delivered each hour to the patient by a medication pump.

The medication order specifies the medication, the volume, and the time period within which the medication is infused into the patient. You calculate the number of drops or the milliliters setting for the medication pump. You'll learn how to perform these calculations in this chapter.

Learning Objectives

➤ Understanding I.V. therapy
➤ Reading the I.V. medication order

➤ The drip rate formula

➤ Calculating the drip rate

➤ The pump rate formula

➤ Calculating the pump rate

➤ Calculating how much longer the I.V. will run

Key Words

Drip rate

Drip factor

Infusion time

gtt

Macropdrops

Microdrops

Electronic medication pump

Drip chamber

Roller clamp

Understanding Intravenous Therapy

The primary goal of I.V. therapy is to deliver medication to the patient quickly. The medication is immediately delivered to the blood stream where it circulates throughout the body. There isn't any delay as with an intramuscular injection or with administering medication orally, which requires the medication to be absorbed into the blood stream.

The medication is contained in either a plastic bag or glass bottle. Tubing connects the bag to the lock, which is attached to the patient's vein. The tubing has a **drip chamber** and a **roller clamp**. The drip chamber is a clear cylinder used to view drops of medication from the bag. The roller clamp is used to control the number of drops of medication per minute that enters the tube from the drip chamber. After calculating the **drip rate**, you use the roller clamp to set the drip rate of the I.V.

ELECTRONIC MEDICATION PUMP

The healthcare facility may require that some or all I.V. medications be administered using an **electronic medication pump**. The pump controls the flow of medication that the patient receives.

Tubing is still used to connect the bag to the lock, however, a portion of the tubing is placed within the pump. The pump takes the place of the roller clamp in controlling the rate of medication received by the patient. The roller clamp is totally open when the pump is used.

The delivery rate on the pump is specified in milliliters/hour for a specific length of time. The medication order specifies the number of milliliters and over what period of time it is to be delivered. You must calculate the hourly rate and then enter the rate into the pump.

Reading the Intravenous Medication Order

In addition to the required elements of a medication order (see Chapter 1), there are three components unique to an I.V. Every I.V. order must have these components, otherwise the medication order is invalid and should not be administered.

Intravenous Solution

The physician must tell you the name of this medication. The order might also have the name of medications that must be added to the I.V. solution depending on the physician's course of treatment.

Volume

This is the amount of the solution that the patient is to receive usually specified in milliliters. It is important to realize that the volume specified in the order may be less than the volume specified on the I.V. bag. Therefore, you base your calculation on the volume ordered by the physician and not the volume on the I.V. bag. You will likely to see questions that show both the volume of the bag and the volume ordered. You must decide which volume to use in your calculation.

Infusion Time

This specifies the time period to give the volume of medication to the patient. The time is commonly ordered as half hour or in hours. Sometimes the time can be in minutes such as within a 15 minute period.

THE INTRAVENOUS BAG

The I.V. bag label contains the name of the medication and the volume contained in the I.V. bag. It also contains text that provides details of the solution including the ratio of medication per 100 mL of I.V. fluid. You don't use this ratio in your flow rate calculation.

At the top of the I.V. bag is a lot number and expiration date. The lot number identifies when the solution was produced. The expiration date is similar to the expiration date on other medications that you learned about in Chapter 1. If the solution has expired, then don't use it.

Numbers along the side of the bag are used to measure the volume of solution infused into the patient. Each represents 100 mL.

The Drip Rate Formula

The drip rate formula is used to calculate the number of drops per minute of the medication that the patient is to receive. This is the number of drops that appears in the drip chamber in a minute.

Here's an example of a medication order for I.V. therapy.

1000 mL DSW I.V. in 8 hours

In order to calculate the drip rate, you need to know:

The **drip factor** of the tubing

Total volume

Number of minutes of the infusion

THE DRIP FACTOR

The drip factor is the number of drops that equals 1 mL. The drip factor depends on the tubing that is used for the infusion and is specified on the bag that contains the tubing. The drip factor is written as gtt/mL where **gtt** is the abbreviation for drop.

For example, the bag containing the I.V. tubing might have 10 gtt/mL on the bag. This is the drip factor for the tubing that you use to calculate the drip rate for the I.V. medication. If you don't see a drip factor on the bag, then don't use the tubing.

There are two categories of drip factors. These are **macrodrops** and **microdrops.** Macrodrop tubing typically has 10, 15, or 20 gtt/mL. Microdrop tubing always has 60 gtt/mL as the drip factor.

HINT *If you see macrodrop on the bag, then use 60 gtt/mL as the drip factor. Macropdrop tubing always has the drip factor marked on the bag.*

PARTS OF THE DRIP RATE FORMULA

There are several different formulas that can be used to calculate the drip rate. Here's the formula that is commonly used:

$$X \text{ gtt/min} = \frac{\text{Volume ordered} \times \text{Drip factor}}{\text{Minutes to infuse}}$$

The value for the volume ordered is found on the medication order. The drip factor is on the I.V. bag. The minutes to infuse the medication is also on the medication order, but this is usually stated as hours or half hour.

Calculating the Drip Rate

Let's calculate the drip rate for the following medication order. Assume that you are using macrodrop tubing with a 10 gtt/mL drip factor.

1000 mL D5W I.V. in 8 hours

1. Convert the **infusion time** from 8 hours to minutes because the drip rate is in minutes.

$$480 \text{ minutes} = 8 \text{ hours} \times 60 \text{ minutes}$$

2. Place values into the formula.

$$X \text{ gtt/min} = \frac{1000 \text{ mL} \times 10 \text{ gtt/mL}}{480 \text{ minutes}}$$

3. Calculate the total number of drops in the volume.

$$X \text{ gtt/min} = \frac{10,000 \text{ gtt}}{480 \text{ minutes}}$$

4. Calculate the number of drops per minute.

$$20.833 \text{ gtt/min} = \frac{10000 \text{ gtt}}{480 \text{ minutes}}$$

5. Round to the whole number. Remember these are drops. You can't set the drip rate to a fraction of a drop. Round up if the value is 5 or greater. Round down if the value is less than 5.

21 gtt/min

SETTING THE DRIP RATE

Now that you calculated the drip rate, you must set this rate using the I.V. tubing roller clamp. You do this by adjusting the roller clamp so that the calculated number of drops fall through the drip chamber each minute. This is 21 drops/min in the previous example.

Setting the drip rate can be tricky because you have to keep one eye on the drip chamber and another on the clock. A method used by some nurses makes this a straightforward process. Hold your watch next to the drip chamber so both are in the same view.

HINT Another trick is to calculate the number of drips for less than a minute. Say that the drip rate per minute is 60 gtt. This also means there are 6 gtt per 10 seconds. You need only to see 6 drops within 10 seconds in the drip chamber to set the correct drip rate rather that counting drops for a full minute.

Practice Drill 4.1—the Drip Rate Formula

Calculating the drip factor is straightforward. Try your hand at calculating the drip factor for the following orders:

1. Medication order: 1000 mL normal saline I.V. at 40 mL/hr
   Use tubing with a 15 gtt/mL drip factor

   What is the drip rate?

2. Medication order: 1 L normal saline I.V. over 12 hours
   Use tubing with a 10 gtt/mL drip factor

   What is the drip rate?

3. Medication order: Cefadyl 5 g diluted in 100 mL of normal saline I.V. over a half hour
   Use tubing with a 10 gtt/mL drip factor

   What is the drip rate?

4. Medication order: Gentamycin 2 g diluted in 100 mL of normal saline
   I.V. over 1 hour
   Use tubing with a 15 gtt/mL drip factor

   What is the drip rate?

5. Medication order: 1000 mL normal saline I.V. over 15 hours
   Use tubing with a 15 gtt/mL drip factor

   What is the drip rate?

6. Medication order: 1000 mL of 0.9% of sodium chloride I.V. over
   60 mL/hr
   Use tubing with a 10 gtt/mL drip factor

   What is the drip rate?

7. Medication order: 500 mL Ringers Lactate I.V. over 6 hours
   Use tubing with a 10 gtt/mL drip factor

   What is the drip rate?

8. Medication order: 25 mL normal saline I.V. over 30 minutes
   Use tubing with a 15 gtt/mL drip factor

   What is the drip rate?

9. Medication order: 1000 mL Ringers Lactate I.V. over 5 hours
   Use microdrip tubing

   What is the drip rate?

10. Medication order: 2000 mL of 0.9% of sodium chloride I.V. over
    24 hours
    Use tubing with a 10 gtt/mL drip factor

    What is the drip rate?

Solutions to Practice Drill 4.1—the Drip Rate Formula

1. 60 minutes = 1 hour

$$X \text{ gtt/min} = \frac{40 \text{ mL} \times 15 \text{ gtt/mL}}{60 \text{ minutes}}$$

$$X \text{ gtt/min} = \frac{600 \text{ gtt}}{60 \text{ minutes}}$$

$$= 10 \text{ gtt/min}$$

2. $1000 \text{ mL} = 1 \text{ L} \times 1000$

$720 \text{ minutes} = 12 \text{ hours} \times 60 \text{ minutes}$

$$X \text{ gtt/min} = \frac{1000 \text{ mL} \times 10 \text{ gtt/mL}}{720 \text{ minutes}}$$

$$X \text{ gtt/min} = \frac{10,000 \text{ gtt}}{720 \text{ minutes}}$$

$$= 13.888 \text{ gtt/min}$$

$$= 14 \text{ gtt/min}$$

3. $X \text{ gtt/min} = \dfrac{100 \text{ mL} \times 10 \text{ gtt/mL}}{30 \text{ minutes}}$

$$X \text{ gtt/min} = \frac{1000 \text{ gtt}}{30 \text{ minutes}}$$

$$= 33.333 \text{ gtt/min}$$

$$= 33 \text{ gtt/min}$$

4. $60 \text{ minutes} = 1 \text{ hour}$

$$X \text{ gtt/min} = \frac{100 \text{ mL} \times 15 \text{ gtt/mL}}{60 \text{ minutes}}$$

$$X \text{ gtt/min} = \frac{1500 \text{ gtt}}{60 \text{ minutes}}$$

$$= 25 \text{ gtt/min}$$

5. $900 \text{ minutes} = 15 \text{ hours} \times 60 \text{ minutes}$

$$X \text{ gtt/min} = \frac{1000 \text{ mL} \times 15 \text{ gtt/mL}}{900 \text{ minutes}}$$

$$X \text{ gtt/min} = \frac{15,000 \text{ gtt}}{900 \text{ minutes}}$$

$$= 16.666 \text{ gtt/min}$$

$$= 17 \text{ gtt/min}$$

6. 60 minutes = 1 hour

$$X \text{ gtt/min} = \frac{60 \text{ mL} \times 10 \text{ gtt/mL}}{60 \text{ minutes}}$$

$$X \text{ gtt/min} = \frac{600 \text{ gtt}}{60 \text{ minutes}}$$

$$= 10 \text{ gtt/min}$$

7. 360 minutes = 6 hours × 60 minutes

$$X \text{ gtt/min} = \frac{500 \text{ mL} \times 10 \text{ gtt/mL}}{360 \text{ minutes}}$$

$$X \text{ gtt/min} = \frac{5000 \text{ gtt}}{360 \text{ minutes}}$$

$$= 13.888 \text{ gtt/min}$$

$$= 14 \text{ gtt/min}$$

8. $X \text{ gtt/min} = \dfrac{25 \text{ mL} \times 15 \text{ gtt/mL}}{30 \text{ minutes}}$

$$X \text{ gtt/min} = \frac{375 \text{ gtt}}{30 \text{ minutes}}$$

$$= 12.5 \text{ gtt/min}$$

$$= 13 \text{ gtt/min}$$

9. 300 minutes = 5 hours × 60 minutes

$$X \text{ gtt/min} = \frac{1000 \text{ mL} \times 15 \text{ gtt/mL}}{300 \text{ minutes}}$$

$$X \text{ gtt/min} = \frac{15{,}000 \text{ gtt}}{300 \text{ minutes}}$$

$$= 50 \text{ gtt/min}$$

10. $1440 \text{ minutes} = 24 \text{ hours} \times 60 \text{ minutes}$

$$X \text{ gtt/min} = \frac{2000 \text{ mL} \times 10 \text{ gtt/mL}}{1440 \text{ minutes}}$$

$$X \text{ gtt/min} = \frac{20{,}000 \text{ gtt}}{1440 \text{ minutes}}$$

$$= 13.888 \text{ gtt/min}$$

$$= 14 \text{ gtt/min}$$

Pump Rate

There is a tendency of healthcare facilities to use an electronic medication pump rather than the drip method to control the flow of the medication to the patient. Some medications must be delivered using the electronic medication pump because the flow rate must be accurately metered.

Although there are various kinds of electronic medication pumps used by healthcare facilities, most require three settings. These are the total volume in the bag or bottle, the total length of time of the infusion, and the number of milliliters that are to be infused per hour.

The total volume and the total length of time of the infusion are found in the medication order. You calculate the number of milliliters that are to be infused per hour.

Based on these settings, electronic sensors in the electronic medication pump administer the prescribed dose and stop the flow automatically when the prescribed dose is given. An alarm sounds when the pump stops. This happens whenever the flow stops including if there is a kink in the tube.

THE PUMP RATE FORMULA

The pump rate formula has two components:

Volume: This is the volume in milliliters specified in the medication order:

Time: This is the time in hours specified in the medication order. Pumps will also accept time in minutes.

Here is how to construct the pump rate formula:

$$mL/hr = \frac{volume \text{ mL}}{time \text{ hr}}$$

CALCULATING THE PUMP RATE

Let's say you received the following medication order:

1000 mL normal saline I.V. over 12 hours

An electronic medication pump is available, so you'll need to calculate the volume of normal saline that is to be administered to the patient every hour.

1. Enter the values from the medication order into the formula.

$$\text{mL/hr} = \frac{1000 \text{ mL}}{12 \text{ hr}}$$

2. Calculate the formula.

$$\text{mL/hr} = 83.333$$

3. The pump accepts only whole numbers. Therefore, any decimal values must be rounded. Round up if the decimal value is 5 or greater and round down if the decimal value is less than 5. This is the value that you enter into the pump.

$$\text{mL/hr} = 83 \text{ mL}$$

Practice Drill 4.2—the Pump Rate Formula

Determine the pump setting for each of these orders.

1. Medication order: 1000 mL D5W I.V. over 24 hours
   What is the pump setting?
2. Medication order: 200 mL Lactated Ringers I.V. over 5 hours
   What is the pump setting?
3. Medication order: 1500 mL normal saline I.V. over 12 hours
   What is the pump setting?
4. Medication order: 500 mL D51/2 normal saline I.V. over 8 hours
   What is the pump setting?

5. Medication order: 800 mL ½ normal saline I.V. over 16 hours

What is the pump setting?

6. Medication order: 50 mL D5 normal saline I.V. over 1 hour

What is the pump setting?

7. Medication order: 350 mL D5W I.V. over 4 hours

What is the pump setting?

8. Medication order: 3000 mL normal saline I.V. over 24 hours

What is the pump setting?

9. Medication order: 1500 mL Lactated Ringers I.V. over 16 hours

What is the pump setting?

10. Medication order: 150 mL D51/2 normal saline I.V. over 5 hours

What is the pump setting?

Solutions to Practice Drill 4.2—the Pump Rate Formula

1. $\text{mL/hr} = \dfrac{1000 \text{ mL}}{24 \text{ hours}}$

$\text{mL/hr} = 41.666 \text{ mL}$

$\text{mL/hr} = 42 \text{ mL}$

2. $\text{mL/hr} = \dfrac{200 \text{ mL}}{5 \text{ hours}}$

$\text{mL/hr} = 40 \text{ mL}$

3. $\text{mL/hr} = \dfrac{1500 \text{ mL}}{12 \text{ hours}}$

$\text{mL/hr} = 125 \text{ mL}$

4. $\text{mL/hr} = \dfrac{500 \text{ mL}}{8 \text{ hours}}$

$\text{mL/hr} = 62.5 \text{ mL}$

$\text{mL/hr} = 63 \text{ mL}$

5. $\text{mL/hr} = \dfrac{800 \text{ mL}}{6 \text{ hours}}$

$133.33 = 133 \text{ mL}$

6. $mL/hr = \dfrac{50 \text{ mL}}{1 \text{ hour}}$

$mL/hr = 50 \text{ mL}$

7. $mL/hr = \dfrac{350 \text{ mL}}{4 \text{ hours}}$

$mL/hr = 87.5 \text{ mL}$

$mL/hr = 88 \text{ mL}$

8. $mL/hr = \dfrac{3000 \text{ mL}}{24 \text{ hours}}$

$mL/hr = 125 \text{ mL}$

9. $mL/hr = \dfrac{1500 \text{ mL}}{16 \text{ hours}}$

$mL/hr = 93.75 \text{ mL}$

$mL/hr = 94 \text{ mL}$

10. $mL/hr = \dfrac{150 \text{ mL}}{5 \text{ hours}}$

$mL/hr = 30 \text{ mL}$

Calculating How Much Longer the Intravenous Will Run

You might find that your patient is receiving I.V. medication started by the previous shift and you'll need to know how much time is left before the infusion is completed. This is handy to know so you can schedule your time to care for this and other patients.

You calculate the remaining time by knowing the milliliter per hour setting for the pump and the current volume in the bag.

Here's the formula to use:

$$\text{Time remaining} = \frac{\text{current volume (mL)}}{\text{pump setting (mL)}}$$

Say that your patient has received 150 mL of Lactated Ringers I.V. and the I.V. bag currently has a volume of 100 mL of Lactated Ringers. The pump is set at 30 mL/hr. How much longer does the infusion have to run?

1. Insert the values into the formula.

$$\text{Time remaining} = \frac{50 \text{ mL}}{30 \text{ mL}}$$

2. Divide the current volume by the pump setting.

$$\text{Time remaining} = 1.66 \text{ hours}$$

3. Convert the decimal value to minutes.

$$\text{Minutes} = 60 \text{ minutes} \times 0.66 = 39.6 \text{ minutes} = 40 \text{ minutes}$$

4. Time remaining = 1 hour 40 minutes

HINT *You only need to estimate the time remaining for the infusion.*

Practice Drill 4.3—the Time Remaining Formula

Calculate the remaining infusion time for the following patients. Assume that the I.V. bag contains the total amount that is being infused.

1. 1000 mL D5W I.V. The pump setting is 42 mL. Current volume in the I.V. bag is 750 mL.

   How much time is remaining?

2. 200 mL Lactated Ringers I.V. The pump setting is 40 mL. Current volume in the I.V. bag is 150 mL.

   How much time is remaining?

3. 1500 mL normal saline I.V. The pump setting is 125 mL. Current volume in the I.V. bag is 500 mL.

   How much time is remaining?

4. 500 mL D51/2 normal saline I.V. The pump setting is 63 mL. Current volume in the I.V. bag is 200 mL.

   How much time is remaining?

5. 800 mL ½ normal saline I.V. The pump setting is 50 mL. Current volume in the I.V. bag is 300 mL.

   How much time is remaining?

6. 50 mL D5 normal saline I.V. The pump setting is 50 mL. Current volume in the I.V. bag is 25 mL.

   How much time is remaining?

7. 350 mL D5W I.V. The pump setting is 88 mL. Current volume in the I.V. bag is 150 mL.

   How much time is remaining?

8. 3000 mL normal saline I.V. The pump setting is 125 mL. Current volume in the I.V. bag is 2500 mL.

   How much time is remaining?

9. 1500 mL Lactated Ringers I.V. The pump setting is 94 mL. Current volume in the I.V. bag is 500 mL.

   How much time is remaining?

10. 150 mL D51/2 normal saline I.V. The pump setting is 30 mL. Current volume in the I.V. bag is 25 mL.

    How much time is remaining?

Solutions to Practice Drill 4.3—the Time Remaining Formula

1. Time remaining $= \dfrac{750 \text{ mL}}{42 \text{ mL}}$

   Time remaining = 17.86 hours

   Minutes = 60 minutes $\times$ 0.86 = 51.6 minutes

   Time remaining = 17 hours 52 minutes

2. Time remaining $= \dfrac{150 \text{ mL}}{40 \text{ mL}}$

   Time remaining = 3.75 hours

   Minutes = 60 minutes $\times$ 0.75 = 45 minutes

   Time remaining = 3 hours 45 minutes

3. Time remaining $= \dfrac{500 \text{ mL}}{125 \text{ mL}}$

Time remaining $= 4$ hours

4. Time remaining $= \dfrac{200 \text{ mL}}{63 \text{ mL}}$

Time remaining $= 3.17$ hrs

Minutes $= 60$ minutes $\times 0.17 = 10$ minutes

Time remaining $= 3$ hours 10 minutes

5. Time remaining $= \dfrac{300 \text{ mL}}{50 \text{ mL}}$

Time remaining $= 6$ hours

6. Time remaining $= \dfrac{25 \text{ mL}}{50 \text{ mL}}$

Time remaining $= 0.5$ hours

Minutes $= 60$ minutes $\times 0.5 = 30$ minutes

Time remaining $= 30$ minutes

7. Time remaining $= \dfrac{150 \text{ mL}}{88 \text{ mL}}$

Time remaining $= 1.70$ hours

Minutes $= 60$ minutes $\times 0.70 = 42$ minutes

Time remaining $= 1$ hour 42 minutes

8. Time remaining $= \dfrac{2500 \text{ mL}}{125 \text{ mL}}$

Time remaining $= 20$ hours

9. Time remaining $= \dfrac{500 \text{ mL}}{94 \text{ mL}}$

Time remaining $= 5.31$ hours

Minutes $= 60$ minutes $\times 0.31 = 19$ minutes

Time remaining $= 5$ hours 19 minutes

10. Time remaining $= \dfrac{25 \text{ mL}}{30 \text{ mL}}$

Time remaining $= 0.83$ hours

Minutes $= 60$ minutes $\times 0.83 = 49.8$ minutes

Time remaining $= 50$ minutes

Summary

Intravenous therapy provides a continuous flow of medication to the patient referred to as the infusion. The rate of infusion is controlled by the number of drops of fluid administered to the patient each minute, which is called the drip rate.

The drip rate is calculated using the drip rate formula that uses the drip factor of the I.V. tubing to determine the number of drops per minute of the medication that the patient is to receive. This is set by adjusting the number of drops in the drip chamber using the roller clamp on the I.V. tubing.

Intravenous therapy is also administered using the electronic medication pump. This pump electronically meters a fix number of milliliters per hour. You calculate this value by using the pump rate formula.

There are times when you'll need to know how much longer the infusion will run. You determine this by using the time remaining formula.

Quiz

1. The medication order is for 1000 mL of D5W I.V. that is to be administered over 5 hours. What is the pump setting?

    a.   2 mL

    b.   200 mL

    c.   20 mL

    d.   0.2 mL

2. The medication order is for 1 L of normal saline I.V. that is to be administered over 8 hours. On hand is I.V. tubing with a 10 gtt/mL drip factor. What is the drip setting?

    a.   21 gtt/min

    b.   2.1 gtt/min

c. 210 gtt/min

d. 20 gtt/min

3. The medication order is for Cefadyl 10 g diluted in 200 mL of normal saline I.V. that is to be administered over 4 hours. On hand is I.V. tubing with a 15 gtt/mL drip factor. What is the drip setting?

    a. 12 gtt/min

    b. 12.5 gtt/min

    c. 13 gtt/min

    d. 13.5 gtt/min

4. The medication order is for 200 mL of D5W I.V. that is to be administered over 4 hours. The nurse should set the pump at 50 mL/hr.

    a. True

    b. False

5. Your patient has received 250 mL of normal saline I.V. and the I.V. bag currently has a volume of 75 mL of normal saline. The pump is set at 30 mL/hr. How much longer does the infusion have to run?

    a. 2 hours 35 minutes

    b. 30 minutes

    c. 2 hours

    d. 2 hours 30 minutes

6. The medication order is for 200 mL of D51/2 normal saline I.V. that is to be administered over 7 hours. On hand is I.V. tubing with a 10 gtt/mL drip factor. What is the drip setting?

    a. 5 gtt/min

    b. 5.5 gtt/min

    c. 4 gtt/min

    d. 4.8 gtt/min

7. The medication order is for 3000 mL of ½ normal saline I.V. that is to be administered over 24 hours What is the pump setting?

    a. 124 mL/hr

    b. 120 mL/hr

    c. 125 mL/hr

    d. 126 mL/hr

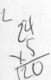

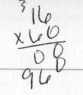

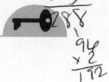

8. The medication order is for 2000 mL of Ringers Lactate I.V. that is to be administered over 16 hours. On hand is I.V. tubing with a 15 gtt/mL drip factor. What is the drip setting?

   a. 31 gtt/min

   b. 31.5 gtt/min

   c. 32 gtt/min

   d. 32.5 gtt/min

$$\frac{2000 \times 15}{960} = \frac{30,000}{960}$$

$$96\overline{)3000.}^{31.7}$$
$$-288$$
$$120$$
$$-96$$
$$240$$
$$-192$$
$$48$$

9. The medication order is for 600 mL of ½ normal saline I.V. that is to be administered over 6 hours. On hand is I.V. tubing with a 10 gtt/mL drip factor. What is the pump setting?

   a. 100 mL/hr

   b. 90 mL/hr

   c. 80 mL/hr

   d. 110 mL/hr

$$\frac{600 \times 10}{360} = \frac{6,000}{360}$$

$$36\overline{)600.}^{16.}$$
$$-36$$
$$240$$
$$-216$$

$$36 \times 6 = 216$$

10. Your patient has received 1500 mL of normal saline I.V. and the I.V. bag currently has a volume of 750 mL of normal saline. The pump is set at 40 mL/hr. How much longer does the infusion have to run?

    a. 18 hours 35 minutes

    b. 10 hours 45 minutes

    c. 8 hours 45 minutes

    d. 18 hours 45 minutes

$$40\overline{)750.}^{18.75}$$
$$-40$$
$$350$$
$$-320$$
$$300$$
$$-280$$
$$200$$

$$40 \times 7 = 280$$

CHAPTER 5

Calculating Pediatric Doses

You were taught in school that pediatric patients are not simply small versions of adult patients. Instead, pediatric patients are at various states of maturity and may lack the capability to adequately metabolize and excrete medications at an adult dose.

The dose of medication for a pediatric patient must be carefully calculated based on the patient's weight because even a small discrepancy can endanger the youngster's health. Furthermore, there is a limit on the amount of a medication that the pediatric patient can receive within 24 hours.

Before administering medication, you'll need to determine the total amount of the medication the youngster has already received and then calculate the dose using the patient's weight. You'll learn how to perform both calculations in this chapter.

Learning Objectives

➤ Calculating pediatric dose

➤ The pediatric dose calculation formula

➤ Calculating the maximum quantity per day

➤ Calculating multiple doses

Key Words

Maximum dose per 24 hours

Dose per kilogram

Dose per day

Loading dose

Converting pounds to kilogram

Calculating Pediatric Doses

The dose of a medication prescribed for an adult is based on a typical adult. The physician may adjust the dose if the patient's condition differs from that of a typical adult because of age or condition of the patient's body. For example, the dose may be decreased for elderly patients or patients with liver disease since the medication is absorbed and metabolized slower than in a typical adult.

In contrast, pediatric medication is prescribed in a dose that is relatively unique for the patient because the prescribed dose is based on the child's weight. The quantity of the medication is written in the medication order per kilogram.

Here's an example:

Elixir of Digoxin 15 mcg

FROM POUNDS TO KILOGRAM

Although some healthcare facilities may record a patient's weight in kilogram, many record the patient's weight in pounds. You'll need to convert the child's weight from pounds to kilograms before calculating the dose.

The conversion process is straightforward if you remember that

$$1 \text{ kg} = 2.2 \text{ lb}$$

Then use the following formula for the conversion.

$$\text{Child's weight (kg)} = \frac{\text{child's weight (lb)}}{2.2 \text{ lb}}$$

Let's say that child weighs 66 lb and you need to convert this weight to kilograms. Here's what to do:

1. Insert values into the formula.

$$\text{Child's weight (kg)} = \frac{66 \text{ lb}}{2.2 \text{ lb}}$$

2. Calculate the formula.

$$30 \text{ kg} = \frac{66 \text{ lb}}{2.2 \text{ lb}}$$

ROUNDING

Expect decimal values when you convert from pounds to kilograms. This isn't a problem as long as you apply the rounding rules that you learned in Chapter 2. Here's what to do:

1. Truncate the kilogram weight to three decimal values.
2. Don't round the kilogram weight.
3. Use the kilogram weight—and its three decimal values—in the pediatric dose calculation.

Suppose the child weighs 50 lb. Insert this value into the formula and calculate. This results in a series of decimal values of 7272727…. Use three decimal values only as shown here:

$$22.727 \text{ kg} = \frac{50 \text{ lb}}{2.2 \text{ lb}}$$

HINT *It is always a good practice to ask another registered nurse to double check your calculations as a precaution.*

The Pediatric Dose Calculation Formula

The pediatric dose calculation formula is very similar to the formula used to calculate an adult dose (see Chapter 2) except the quantity of medication ordered is for 1 kg of the patient's weight. You must first determine the full quantity ordered for the patient and then the dose to administer to the patient.

There are four components of the pediatric dose calculation formula as shown here:

$$\text{Dose} = \frac{\text{orders per kg} \times \text{patient's weight (kg)}}{\text{on hand}} \times \text{quantity on hand}$$

CALCULATING USING THE FORMULA

Let's calculate the dose for Elixir of Digoxin 15 mcg/kg. The patient weighs 66 lb. Previously in this chapter ("From Pounds to Kilogram") the patient's weight was converted to 30 kg. The medication label reads 50 mcg/mL.

1. Insert values into the formula.

$$\text{Dose} = \frac{15 \text{ mcg/kg} \times 30 \text{ kg}}{50 \text{ mcg}} \times 1 \text{ mL}$$

2. Calculate the full quantity ordered by multiplying the quantity per kilogram by the patient's weight.

$$\text{Dose} = \frac{450 \text{ mcg}}{50 \text{ mcg}} \times 1 \text{ mL}$$

3. Calculate the dose as you would an adult dose (see Chapter 2).

$$\text{Dose} = 9 \text{ mcg} \times 1 \text{ mL}$$

$$\text{Dose} = 9 \text{ mcg}$$

Practice Drill 5.1—the Pediatric Dose Calculation Formula

Try your hand at calculating the following doses. Remember to convert the patient's weight from pounds to kilograms before proceeding with the calculation.

1. Medication order: Benadryl 10 mg/kg
   The patient weighs 26 lb.
   Medication label: Benadryl 125 mg/5 mL

   How many milliliters will be administered to the patient?

2. Medication order: Benylin 5 mg/kg
   The patient weighs 44 lb.
   Medication label: Benylin 50 mg per tablet

   How many tablets will be administered to the patient?

3. Medication order: Lithostat 15 mg/kg
   The patient weighs 70 lb.
   Medication label: Lithostat 250 mg per tablet

   How many tablets will be administered to the patient?

4. Medication order: Zovirax 5 mg/kg
   The patient weighs 30 lb.
   Medication label: Zovirax 25 mg/mL

   How many milliliters will be administered to the patient?

5. Medication order: Ampicillin 12.5 mg/kg
   The patient weighs 40 lb.
   Medication label: Ampicillin 100 mg/mL

   How many milliliters will be administered to the patient?

6. Medication order: Zofran 150 mcg/kg
   The patient weighs 65 lb.
   Medication label: Zofran 2000 mcg/mL

   How many milliliters will be administered to the patient?

7. Medication order: Dilantin 1 mg/kg
   The patient weighs 66 lb.
   Medication label: Dilantin 15 mg/capsule

   How many milliliters will be administered to the patient?

8. Medication order: Amoxicillin 10 mg/kg
   The patient weighs 30 lb.
   Medication label: Amoxicillin 125 mg/5 mL

   How many milliliters will be administered to the patient?

9. Medication order: Celocin 6.25 mg/kg
   The patient weighs 45 lb.
   Medication label: Celocin 75 mg/5 mL

   How many milliliters will be administered to the patient?

10. Medication order: Cephalexin 15 mg/kg
    The patient weighs 45 lb.
    Medication label: Cephalexin 125 mg/5 mL

    How many milliliters will be administered to the patient?

Solutions to Practice Drill 5.1—the Pediatric Dose Calculation Formula

1. $11.818 \text{ kg} = \dfrac{26 \text{ lb}}{2.2 \text{ lb}}$

   $\text{Dose} = \dfrac{10 \text{ mg} \times 11.818 \text{ kg}}{125 \text{ mg}} \times 5 \text{ mL}$

   $\text{Dose} = \dfrac{118.18 \text{ mg}}{125 \text{ mg}} \times 5 \text{ mL}$

   $\text{Dose} = 0.945 \times 5 \text{ mL}$

   $\text{Dose} = 4.727 \text{ mL}$

   $\text{Dose} = 4.7 \text{ mL}$

2. $20 \text{ kg} = \dfrac{44 \text{ lb}}{2.2 \text{ lb}}$

   $\text{Dose} = \dfrac{5 \text{ mg} \times 20 \text{ kg}}{50 \text{ mg}} \times 1 \text{ tablet}$

   $\text{Dose} = \dfrac{100 \text{ mg}}{50 \text{ mg}} \times 1 \text{ tablet}$

   $\text{Dose} = 2 \times 1 \text{ tablet}$

   $\text{Dose} = 2 \text{ tablets}$

3. $31.818 \text{ kg} = \dfrac{70 \text{ lb}}{2.2 \text{ lb}}$

$\text{Dose} = \dfrac{15 \text{ mg} \times 31.818 \text{ kg}}{250 \text{ mg}} \times 1 \text{ tablet}$

$\text{Dose} = \dfrac{477.27 \text{ mg}}{250 \text{ mg}} \times 1 \text{ tablet}$

$\text{Dose} = 1.909 \text{ mg}$

$\text{Dose} = 1.909 \times 1 \text{ tablet}$

$\text{Dose} = 2 \text{ tablets}$

4. $13.636 \text{ kg} = \dfrac{30 \text{ lb}}{2.2 \text{ lb}}$

$\text{Dose} = \dfrac{5 \text{ mg} \times 13.636 \text{ kg}}{25 \text{ mg}} \times 1 \text{ mL}$

$\text{Dose} = \dfrac{68.18 \text{ mg}}{25 \text{ mg}} \times 1 \text{ mL}$

$\text{Dose} = 2.727 \text{ mg}$

$\text{Dose} = 2.727 \text{ mg} \times 1 \text{ mL}$

$\text{Dose} = 2.7 \text{ mL}$

5. $18.181 \text{ kg} = \dfrac{40 \text{ lb}}{2.2 \text{ lb}}$

$\text{Dose} = \dfrac{12.5 \text{ mg} \times 18.181 \text{ kg}}{100 \text{ mg}} \times 1 \text{ mL}$

$\text{Dose} = \dfrac{227.262 \text{ mg}}{100 \text{ mg}} \times 1 \text{ mL}$

$\text{Dose} = 2.272 \text{ mg}$

$\text{Dose} = 2.272 \text{ mg} \times 1 \text{ mL}$

$\text{Dose} = 2.3 \text{ mL}$

6. $29.545 \text{ kg} = \dfrac{65 \text{ lb}}{2.2 \text{ lb}}$

$$\text{Dose} = \dfrac{150 \text{ mcg} \times 29.545 \text{ kg}}{2000 \text{ mcg}} \times 1 \text{ mL}$$

$$\text{Dose} = \dfrac{4431.75 \text{ mcg}}{2000 \text{ mcg}} \times 1 \text{ mL}$$

$$\text{Dose} = 2.215 \text{ mcg}$$

$$\text{Dose} = 2.215 \text{ mcg} \times 1 \text{ mL}$$

$$\text{Dose} = 2.2 \text{ mL}$$

7. $30 \text{ kg} = \dfrac{66 \text{ lb}}{2.2 \text{ lb}}$

$$\text{Dose} = \dfrac{1 \text{ mg} \times 30 \text{ kg}}{15 \text{ mg}} \times 1 \text{ capsule}$$

$$\text{Dose} = \dfrac{30 \text{ mg}}{15 \text{ mg}} \times 1 \text{ capsule}$$

$$\text{Dose} = 2 \text{ mg} \times 1 \text{ capsule}$$

$$\text{Dose} = 2 \text{ capsules}$$

8. $13.636 \text{ kg} = \dfrac{30 \text{ lb}}{2.2 \text{ lb}}$

$$\text{Dose} = \dfrac{10 \text{ mg} \times 13.636 \text{ kg}}{125 \text{ mg}} \times 5 \text{ mL}$$

$$\text{Dose} = \dfrac{136.36 \text{ mg}}{125 \text{ mg}} \times 5 \text{ mL}$$

$$\text{Dose} = 1.090 \text{ mg} \times 5 \text{ mL}$$

$$\text{Dose} = 5.454 \text{ mL}$$

$$\text{Dose} = 5.5 \text{ mL}$$

9. $20.454 \text{ kg} = \dfrac{45 \text{ lb}}{2.2 \text{ lb}}$

$\text{Dose} = \dfrac{6.25 \text{ mg} \times 20.454 \text{ kg}}{75 \text{ mg}} \times 5 \text{ mL}$

$\text{Dose} = \dfrac{127.837 \text{ mg}}{75 \text{ mg}} \times 5 \text{ mL}$

$\text{Dose} = 1.704 \text{ mg} \times 5 \text{ mL}$

$\text{Dose} = 8.522 \text{ mL}$

$\text{Dose} = 8.5 \text{ mL}$

10. $20.454 \text{ kg} = \dfrac{45 \text{ lb}}{2.2 \text{ lb}}$

$\text{Dose} = \dfrac{15 \text{ mg} \times 20.454 \text{ kg}}{125 \text{ mg}} \times 5 \text{ mL}$

$\text{Dose} = \dfrac{306.81 \text{ mg}}{125 \text{ mg}} \times 5 \text{ mL}$

$\text{Dose} = 2.454 \text{ mg} \times 5 \text{ mL}$

$\text{Dose} = 12.274 \text{ mL}$

$\text{Dose} = 12 \text{ mL}$

Calculating the Maximum Quantity per Day

Drug manufacturers determine the maximum quantity of a medication that a child can receive within a 24-hour period. A medication order that exceeds the allowable amount must be questioned because the physician may not be aware of the amount of the medication that the child has already received.

Before administering medication to the child, you must determine the maximum quantity of the medication that is permissible within a 24-hour period. You'll find this information in a drug guide on the unit.

Next, review the Medication Administration Record (see Chapter 1) and calculate the total amount of the medication that the child received within the last 24 hours.

Next, calculate the dose you plan to administer to the child. Add this amount to the total the child received so far within 24 hours and compare the result to the maximum allowable from the drug guide.

If child hasn't received the maximum amount, then administer the next dose, otherwise don't administer the medication. Report your findings to the physician.

Calculating Multiple Doses

Typically the patient receives multiple doses of the same medication over course of a day. The physician may order a loading dose first followed by a series of maintenance doses. The loading dose is a high dose to deliver a larger amount of medication to the patient quickly. A maintenance dose is a lower dose designed to maintain the therapeutic level of the medication.

The medication order for the maintenance doses usually specifies a daily quantity of medication that is to be administered multiple times during the day. For example, the physician might write

Ampicillin 50 mg/kg per day q6h

You need to calculate the dose that is to be administered every 6 hours.

THE MULTIPLE DOSE FORMULA

The multiple dose formula is very similar to the pediatric dose calculation formula. Both formulas result in a dose; however, the multiple dose formula results in the dose for the entire 24-hour period and therefore must be divided by the number of doses specified in the medication order.

Here is the multiple dose formula:

$$\text{Dose / day} = \frac{\text{orders/kg} \times \text{patient's weight (kg)}}{\text{on hand}} \times \text{quantity on hand}$$

$$\text{Dose} = \frac{\text{dose/day}}{\text{ordered number of doses}}$$

CALCULATING USING THE FORMULA

Let's calculate the dose for Ampicillin 50 mg/kg·day every 6 hours. The patient weighs 30 lb. Previously in this chapter ("From Pounds to Kilogram") the patient's weight was converted to 13.636 kg. The medication label reads 100 mg/mL.

1. Insert values into the formula.

$$\text{Dose per day} = \frac{50 \text{ mg} \times 13.636 \text{ kg}}{100 \text{ mg}} \times 1 \text{ mL}$$

2. Calculate the **dose per day.**

$$\text{Dose per day} = \frac{50 \text{ mg} \times 13.636 \text{ kg}}{100 \text{ mg}} \times 1 \text{ mL}$$

$$\text{Dose per day} = \frac{681.8 \text{ mg}}{100 \text{ mg}} \times 1 \text{ mL}$$

$$\text{Dose per day} = 6.818 \text{ mg} \times 1 \text{ mL}$$

$$\text{Dose per day} = 6.8 \text{ mL}$$

3. Insert values into the formula.

$$\text{Dose} = \frac{6.8 \text{ mL}}{4 \text{ doses ordered}}$$

4. Calculate the dose.

$$\text{Dose} = 1.7 \text{ mL}$$

HINT *Table 1.3 in Chapter 1 contains abbreviations used to specify the frequency of when to administer a medication to a patient. If order specifies the frequency in hours such as every 6 hours (q6h), divide the 24 hours by the frequency to identify the number of doses that must be administered to the patient. For example,*

$$4 \text{ doses} = \frac{24 \text{ hours}}{6}$$

Practice Drill 5.2—the Multidose Calculation Formula

Calculate the dose for these multidose orders. Be sure to calculate the patient's weight in pounds before calculating the dose per day.

1. Medication order: Benadryl 30 mg/kg/day q6h
   The patient weighs 66 lb.
   Medication label: Benadryl 125 mg/5 mL

   How many milliliters per dose will be administered to the patient?

2. Medication order: Benylin 25 mg/kg/day q3h
   The patient weighs 55 lb.
   Medication label: Benylin 25 mg/mL

   How many milliliters per dose will be administered to the patient?

3. Medication order: Lithostat 120 mg/kg/day q4h
   The patient weighs 110 lb.
   Medication label: Lithostat 250 mg/mL

   How many milliliters per dose will be administered to the patient?

4. Medication order: Zovirax 5 mg/kg/day q12h
   The patient weighs 55 lb.
   Medication label: Zovirax 25 mg per tablet

   How many tablets per dose will be administered to the patient?

5. Medication order: Ampicillin 15 mg/kg/day q8/h
   The patient weighs 44 lb.
   Medication label: Ampicillin 100 mg/mL

   How many milliliters per dose will be administered to the patient?

6. Medication order: Zofran 120 mg/kg/day q6h
   The patient weighs 33 lb.
   Medication label: Zofran 200 mg/mL

   How many milliliters per dose will be administered to the patient?

7. Medication order: Dilantin 30 mg/kg/day q8h
   The patient weighs 55 lb.
   Medication label: Dilantin 40 mg/mL

   How many milliliters per dose will be administered to the patient?

8. Medication order: Amoxicillin 10 mg/kg/day q6h
   The patient weighs 44 lb.
   Medication label: Amoxicillin 125 mg/5 mL

   How many milliliters per dose will be administered to the patient?

9. Medication order: Celocin 45 mg/kg/day q4h
   The patient weighs 110 lb.
   Medication label: Celocin 125 mg/5 mL

   How many milliliters per dose will be administered to the patient?

10. Medication order: Cephalexin 15 mg/kg/day q6h
    The patient weighs 132 lb.
    Medication label: Cephalexin 125 mg/5 mL

    How many milliliters per dose will be administered to the patient?

Solutions to Practice Drill 5.2—the Multidose Calculation Formula

1.
$$4 \text{ doses} = \frac{24 \text{ hours}}{6}$$

$$30 \text{ kg} = \frac{66 \text{ lb}}{2.2 \text{ lb}}$$

$$\text{Dose per day} = \frac{30 \text{ mg} \times 30 \text{ kg}}{125 \text{ mg}} \times 5 \text{ mL}$$

$$= \frac{900 \text{ mg}}{125 \text{ mg}} \times 5 \text{ mL}$$

$$\text{Dose per day} = 7.2 \text{ mg} \times 5 \text{ mL}$$

$$\text{Dose per day} = 36 \text{ mL}$$

$$\text{Per dose} = \frac{36 \text{ mL}}{4 \text{ doses}}$$

$$\text{Per dose} = 9 \text{ mL}$$

2.
$$8 \text{ doses} = \frac{24 \text{ hours}}{3}$$

$$25 \text{ kg} = \frac{55 \text{ lb}}{2.2 \text{ lb}}$$

$$\text{Dose per day} = \frac{50 \text{ mg} \times 25 \text{ kg}}{25 \text{ mg}} \times 1 \text{ mL}$$

$$= \frac{1250 \text{ mg}}{25 \text{ mg}} \times 1 \text{ mL}$$

$$\text{Dose per day} = 50 \text{ mg} \times 1 \text{ mL}$$

$$\text{Dose per day} = 50 \text{ mL}$$

$$\text{Per dose} = \frac{50 \text{ mL}}{8 \text{ doses}}$$

$$\text{Per dose} = 6.25 \text{ mL}$$

3.
$$6 \text{ doses} = \frac{24 \text{ hours}}{4}$$

$$50 \text{ kg} = \frac{110 \text{ lb}}{2.2 \text{ lb}}$$

$$\text{Dose per day} = \frac{120 \text{ mg} \times 50 \text{ kg}}{250 \text{ mg}} \times 1 \text{ mL}$$

$$= \frac{6000 \text{ mg}}{250 \text{ mg}} \times 1 \text{ mL}$$

$$\text{Dose per day} = 24 \text{ mg} \times 1 \text{ mL}$$

$$\text{Dose per day} = 24 \text{ mL}$$

$$\text{Per dose} = \frac{24 \text{ mL}}{6 \text{ doses}}$$

$$\text{Per dose} = 4 \text{ mL}$$

4.
$$2 \text{ doses} = \frac{24 \text{ hours}}{12}$$

$$25 \text{ kg} = \frac{55 \text{ lb}}{2.2 \text{ lb}}$$

$$\text{Dose per day} = \frac{5 \text{ mg} \times 25 \text{ kg}}{25 \text{ mg}} \times 1 \text{ tablet}$$

$$= \frac{125 \text{ mg}}{25 \text{ mg}} \times 1 \text{ tablet}$$

$$\text{Dose per day} = 5 \text{ mg} \times 1 \text{ tablet}$$

$$\text{Dose per day} = 5 \text{ tablets}$$

$$\text{Per dose} = \frac{5 \text{ tablets}}{2 \text{ doses}}$$

$$\text{Per dose} = 2.5 \text{ tablets}$$

5.$\qquad 3 \text{ doses} = \dfrac{24 \text{ hours}}{8}$

$$20 \text{ kg} = \dfrac{44 \text{ lb}}{2.2 \text{ lb}}$$

$$\text{Dose per day} = \dfrac{15 \text{ mg} \times 20 \text{ kg}}{100 \text{ mg}} \times 1 \text{ mL}$$

$$= \dfrac{300 \text{ mg}}{100 \text{ mg}} \times 1 \text{ mL}$$

$$\text{Dose per day} = 3 \text{ mg} \times 1 \text{ mL}$$

$$\text{Dose per day} = 3 \text{ mL}$$

$$\text{Per dose} = \dfrac{3 \text{ mL}}{3 \text{ doses}}$$

$$\text{Per dose} = 1 \text{ mL}$$

6.$\qquad 4 \text{ doses} = \dfrac{24 \text{ hours}}{6}$

$$15 \text{ kg} = \dfrac{33 \text{ lb}}{2.2 \text{ lb}}$$

$$\text{Dose per day} = \dfrac{120 \text{ mg} \times 15 \text{ kg}}{200 \text{ mg}} \times 1 \text{ mL}$$

$$= \dfrac{1800 \text{ mg}}{200 \text{ mg}} \times 1 \text{ mL}$$

$$\text{Dose per day} = 9 \text{ mg} \times 1 \text{ mL}$$

$$\text{Dose per day} = 9 \text{ mL}$$

$$\text{Per dose} = \dfrac{9 \text{ mL}}{4 \text{ doses}}$$

$$\text{Per dose} = 2.25 \text{ mL}$$

7. $$3 \text{ doses} = \frac{24 \text{ hours}}{8}$$

$$25 \text{ kg} = \frac{55 \text{ lb}}{2.2 \text{ lb}}$$

$$\text{Dose per day} = \frac{30 \text{ mg} \times 25 \text{ kg}}{40 \text{ mg}} \times 1 \text{ mL}$$

$$= \frac{750 \text{ mg}}{40 \text{ mg}} \times 1 \text{ mL}$$

$$\text{Dose per day} = 18.75 \text{ mg} \times 1 \text{ mL}$$

$$\text{Dose per day} = 18.75 \text{ mL}$$

$$\text{Per dose} = \frac{18.75 \text{ mL}}{3 \text{ doses}}$$

$$\text{Per dose} = 6.25 \text{ mL}$$

8. $$4 \text{ doses} = \frac{24 \text{ hours}}{6}$$

$$20 \text{ kg} = \frac{44 \text{ lb}}{2.2 \text{ lb}}$$

$$\text{Dose per day} = \frac{10 \text{ mg} \times 20 \text{ kg}}{125 \text{ mg}} \times 5 \text{ mL}$$

$$= \frac{200 \text{ mg}}{125 \text{ mg}} \times 5 \text{ mL}$$

$$\text{Dose per day} = 1.6 \text{ mg} \times 5 \text{ mL}$$

$$\text{Dose per day} = 8 \text{ mL}$$

$$\text{Per dose} = \frac{8 \text{ mL}}{4 \text{ doses}}$$

$$\text{Per dose} = 2 \text{ mL}$$

9. $6 \text{ doses} = \dfrac{24 \text{ hours}}{4}$

$50 \text{ kg} = \dfrac{110 \text{ lb}}{2.2 \text{ lb}}$

$\text{Dose per day} = \dfrac{45 \text{ mg} \times 50 \text{ kg}}{125 \text{ mg}} \times 5 \text{ mL}$

$= \dfrac{2250 \text{ mg}}{125 \text{ mg}} \times 5 \text{ mL}$

$\text{Dose per day} = 18 \text{ mg} \times 5 \text{ mL}$

$\text{Dose per day} = 90 \text{ mL}$

$\text{Per dose} = \dfrac{90 \text{ mL}}{6 \text{ doses}}$

$\text{Per dose} = 15 \text{ mL}$

10. $4 \text{ doses} = \dfrac{24 \text{ hours}}{6}$

$60 \text{ kg} = \dfrac{132 \text{ lb}}{2.2 \text{ lb}}$

$\text{Dose per day} = \dfrac{15 \text{ mg} \times 60 \text{ kg}}{125 \text{ mg}} \times 5 \text{ mL}$

$= \dfrac{900 \text{ mg}}{125 \text{ mg}} \times 5 \text{ mL}$

$\text{Dose per day} = 7.2 \text{ mg} \times 5 \text{ mL}$

$\text{Dose per day} = 36 \text{ mL}$

$\text{Per dose} = \dfrac{36 \text{ mL}}{4 \text{ doses}}$

$\text{Per dose} = 9 \text{ mL}$

Summary

Medication for pediatric patient is prescribed by **dose per kilogram** of the patient's weight. Therefore you'll need to convert the patient's weight in pounds to kilograms before the dose to administer to the patient.

Before administering medication to the child you must determine the maximum quantity of medication that is permissible within a 24-hour period, which you'll find in the drug guide. Hold the dose and contact the physician if the next dose exceeds the maximum allowed quantity of the medication.

A physician will frequently order a quantity of medication that is to be administered throughout the day. You must calculate the quantity of each dose that you administer to the patient.

Quiz

1. The physician ordered Digoxin 15 mcg/kg. The patient weighs 44 lb. The medication label reads 75 mcg/mL. What dose will you administer to the patient?

   a. 4 mL

   b. 400 mL

   c. 40 mL

   d. 0.4 mL

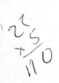

2. The physician ordered Dilantin 45 mg/kg · day q4h. The patient weighs 110 lb. The medication label reads 125 mg/5 mL. What dose will you administer to the patient?

   a. 21 mL

   b. 1.5 mL

   c. 15 mL

   d. 20 mL

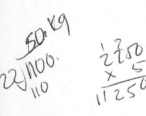

3. The physician ordered Ampicillin 5 mg/kg. The patient weighs 55 lb. The medication label reads 25 mg/mL. What dose will you administer to the patient?

   a. 0.5 mL

   b. 5 mL

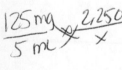
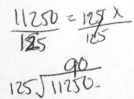

c. 50 mL

    d. 0.05 mL

4. The physician ordered Zofran 120 mg/kg. The patient weighs 33 lb. The medication label reads 200 mg/mL. You will administer 9 mL to the patient.

    a. True

    b. False

5. The physician ordered Lithostat 15 mg/kg. The patient weighs 44 lb. The medication label reads 100 mg/mL. What dose will you administer to the patient?

    a. 5 mL

    b. 4 mL

    c. 3 mL

    d. 2 mL

6. The physician ordered Celocin 10 mg/kg · day q6h. The patient weighs 44 lb. The medication label reads 125 mg/mL. What dose will you administer to the patient?

    a. 0.5 mL

    b. 0.2 mL

    c. 0.4 mL

    d. 0.3 mL

7. The physician ordered Benylin 120 mg/kg. The patient weighs 33 lb. The medication label reads 200 mg/mL. What dose will you administer to the patient?

    a. 1 mL

    b. 1.9 mL

    c. 0.9 mL

    d. 9 mL

8. The physician ordered Benadryl 15 mg/kg. The patient weighs 132 lb. The medication label reads 125 mg/mL. What dose will you administer to the patient?

    a. 7.2 mL

    b. 7 mL

c. 8 mL

     d. 0.72 mL

9. The physician ordered Ampicillin 30 mg/kg. The patient weighs 22 lb. The medication label reads 125 mg/mL. What dose will you administer to the patient?

     a. 2 mL

     b. 0.24 mL

     c. 24 mL

     d. 2.4 mL

10. The physician ordered Zovirax 10 mg/kg. The patient weighs 77 lb. The medication label reads 100 mg/mL. What dose will you administer to the patient?

     a. 3.5 mL

     b. 3 mL

     c. 4 mL

     d. 4.3 mL

CHAPTER 6

Calculating Heparin Dose

Heparin is an anticoagulant (prevents the formation of blood clots) that is prescribed to patients who have venous thromboembolism, unstable angina, acute myocardial infarction, and other conditions that are associated with blood clots. Heparin is administered as a subcutaneous (s.c.) injection or administered intravenously and is also used to flush a Hep-Lock that connects intravenous (I.V.) tubing to the patient's vein.

So far nearly all dosages that you calculated throughout this book used metric units—milligrams, micrograms, and milliliters. Heparin is different and is measured in USP units (U), which is a standard set by the United States Pharmacopeial Convention Inc.

In this chapter you'll learn how to read a medication order for heparin and calculate the proper dose to administer to your patient.

Learning Objectives

➤ A closer look at heparin

➤ Calculating a heparin dose

➤ The heparin dose calculation formula

➤ Be prepared for a different type of heparin question

➤ The heparin subcutaneous formula

Key Words

Partial thromboplastin time (PTT)

Therapeutic level

Anticoagulant

Protamine

Anaphylactic reaction

A Closer Look at Heparin

Heparin prevents blood from clotting, which is the goal if the patient is at risk for blood clots, but too much heparin can lead to excessive bleeding even from a slight injury. Therefore it is important to maintain a **therapeutic level** of heparin at all times.

The therapeutic level is a range that is measured using the **partial thromboplastin time** (PTT) test. A baseline PTT is taken before heparin is administered. The physician uses the test results to determine the dose to prescribe to the patient. Another PTT test is performed 4 hours to 12 hours after the heparin is administered depending on the healthcare facility's policy. Based on the test results, the physician determines if any adjustments must be made to the dose.

If the patient has minor bleeding, then heparin is stopped and vital signs and complete blood count (CBC) is taken. However, if the patient experiences major bleeding, then the physician will likely to order **Protamine** to reverse the effect of heparin. Protamine can cause an **anaphylactic reaction.**

HINT *Heparin has a high potential for injuring the patient, so it is a good idea to have another registered nurse confirm your heparin calculation and double check your setting of the heparin I.V.*

Calculating a Heparin Dose

Heparin-administered I.V. is ordered as units per hour(s). The pharmacy delivers heparin mixed with I.V. fluid such as normal saline or D5W. You must calculate the number of milliliters per hour to administer to your patient.

Here's an example of a heparin order:

Heparin 800U per hour

The Heparin Dose Calculation Formula

The heparin calculation is a two-step process. First you must calculate number of heparin units in a milliliter of I.V. fluids. And then calculate the number of milliliters to administer per hour to the patient.

Here's the heparin formula

1. Calculate the number of heparin units in a milliliter

$$\text{Heparin (U/mL)} = \frac{\text{on hand heparin (U)}}{\text{on hand (mL)}}$$

2. Calculate the number of milliliters to administer per hour

$$\text{Dose (mL/hr)} = \frac{\text{ordered heparin (U)}}{\text{heparin (U/hr)}}$$

CALCULATING USING THE FORMULA

Let's calculate the dose for heparin 800 U/hr. On hand is 25,000 U of heparin in 250 mL of D5W.

1. Insert the values in the first step of calculation.

$$\text{Heparin (U/mL)} = \frac{25000\ \text{(U)}}{250\ \text{(mL)}}$$

2. Calculate the number of heparin units in a milliliter.

$$\text{Heparin (U/mL)} = 100\ \text{U}$$

3. Insert values in the second step of calculation.

$$\text{Dose (mL/hr)} = \frac{800 \text{ U}}{100 \text{ U}}$$

4. Calculate the number of milliliters per hour to administer to the patient.

$$\text{Dose (mL/hr)} = 8 \text{ mL/hr}$$

Practice Drill 6.1—the Heparin Dose Calculation Formula

Calculate the following doses:

1. Medication order: heparin 600 U/hr
   Medication label: 20,000 U heparin in 1000 mL normal saline

   How many milliliters will be administered to the patient per hour?

2. Medication order: heparin 400 U/hr
   Medication label: 20,000 U heparin in 2000 mL normal saline

   How many milliliters will be administered to the patient per hour?

3. Medication order: heparin 200 U/hr
   Medication label: 25,000 U heparin in 500 mL D5W

   How many milliliters will be administered to the patient per hour?

4. Medication order: heparin 250 U/hr
   Medication label: 25,000 U heparin in 1000 mL D5W

   How many milliliters will be administered to the patient per hour?

5. Medication order: heparin 75 U/hr
   Medication label: 25,000 U heparin in 2000 mL normal saline

   How many milliliters will be administered to the patient per hour?

6. Medication order: heparin 300 U/hr
   Medication label: 20,000 U heparin in 1000 mL D5W

   How many milliliters will be administered to the patient per hour?

7. Medication order: heparin 800 U/hr
   Medication label: 10,000 U heparin in 500 mL normal saline

   How many milliliters will be administered to the patient per hour?

8. Medication order: heparin 400 U/hr
   Medication label: 25,000 U heparin in 2000 mL D5W

   How many milliliters will be administered to the patient per hour?

9. Medication order: heparin 700 U/hr
   Medication label: 25,000 U heparin in 250 mL normal saline

   How many milliliters will be administered to the patient per hour?

10. Medication order: heparin 300 U/hr
    Medication label: 25,000 U heparin in 250 mL D5W

    How many milliliters will be administered to the patient per hour?

Solutions to Practice Drill 6.1—the Heparin Dose Calculation Formula

1. $\text{Heparin (U/mL)} = \dfrac{20{,}000 \text{ U}}{1000 \text{ mL}}$

   $\text{Dose (mL/hr)} = \dfrac{600 \text{ U}}{20 \text{ U}}$

   $\text{Dose (mL/hr)} = 30 \text{ mL}$

2. $\text{Heparin (U/mL)} = \dfrac{20{,}000 \text{ U}}{2000 \text{ mL}}$

   $\text{Dose (mL/hr)} = \dfrac{400 \text{ U}}{10 \text{ U}}$

   $\text{Dose (mL/hr)} = 40 \text{ mL}$

3. $\text{Heparin (U/mL)} = \dfrac{25{,}000 \text{ U}}{500 \text{ mL}}$

   $\text{Dose (mL/hr)} = \dfrac{200 \text{ U}}{50 \text{ U}}$

   $\text{Dose (mL/hr)} = 4 \text{ mL}$

4. $\text{Heparin (U/mL)} = \dfrac{25{,}000 \text{ U}}{1000 \text{ mL}}$

   $\text{Dose (mL/hr)} = \dfrac{250 \text{ U}}{25 \text{ U}}$

   $\text{Dose (mL/hr)} = 10 \text{ mL}$

5. $\text{Heparin (U/mL)} = \dfrac{25{,}000 \text{ U}}{2000 \text{ mL}}$

$\text{Dose (mL/hr)} = \dfrac{75 \text{ U}}{12.5 \text{ U}}$

$\text{Dose (mL/hr)} = 6 \text{ mL}$

6. $\text{Heparin (U/mL)} = \dfrac{20{,}000 \text{ U}}{1000 \text{ mL}}$

$\text{Dose (mL/hr)} = \dfrac{300 \text{ U}}{20 \text{ U}}$

$\text{Dose (mL/hr)} = 15 \text{ mL}$

7. $\text{Heparin (U/mL)} = \dfrac{10{,}000 \text{ U}}{500 \text{ mL}}$

$\text{Dose (mL/hr)} = \dfrac{800 \text{ U}}{20 \text{ U}}$

$\text{Dose (mL/hr)} = 40 \text{ mL}$

8. $\text{Heparin (U/mL)} = \dfrac{25{,}000 \text{ U}}{2000 \text{ mL}}$

$\text{Dose (mL/hr)} = \dfrac{400 \text{ U}}{12.5 \text{ U}}$

$\text{Dose (mL/hr)} = 32 \text{ mL}$

9. $\text{Heparin (U/mL)} = \dfrac{25{,}000 \text{ U}}{250 \text{ mL}}$

$\text{Dose (mL/hr)} = \dfrac{700 \text{ U}}{100 \text{ U}}$

$\text{Dose (mL/hr)} = 7 \text{ mL}$

10. $\text{Heparin (U/mL)} = \dfrac{25{,}000 \text{ U}}{250 \text{ mL}}$

$\text{Dose (mL/hr)} = \dfrac{300 \text{ U}}{100 \text{ U}}$

$\text{Dose (mL/hr)} = 3 \text{ mL}$

Be Prepared for Different Type of Heparin Questions

Don't be surprised if you are given the infusion rate on an exam and then asked to calculate the number of unit of heparin that the patient received. For example, you see this order on the exam written as:

25,000 U heparin in 250 cc of D5W infused at 7 mL/U

The formula used to calculate the units of heparin that the patient received is a variation of heparin calculation formula. Here it is:

$$\text{Heparin (U/mL)} = \frac{\text{ordered (U)}}{\text{ordered (mL)}}$$

$$\text{Heparin (U)} = \text{heparin (U/mL)} \times \text{ordered (mL/hr)}$$

Insert the values specified in the order into the formula and then calculate as shown here:

$$\text{Heparin (U/mL)} = \frac{25,000 \text{ U}}{250 \text{ mL}}$$

$$\text{Heparin (U)} = 100 \text{ U} \times 7 \text{ mL/hr}$$

$$\text{Heparin (U)} = 700 \text{ U}$$

Check your answer by using the heparin calculation formula. Assume that the physician ordered 700 U of heparin for the patient and that you have on hand 25,000 U of heparin in 250 mL of D5W. Insert these values into the heparin calculation formula and calculate the dose per hour. The dose per hour should be the same as dose per hour specified in the original order.

$$\text{Heparin (U/mL)} = \frac{25,000 \text{ U}}{250 \text{ mL}}$$

$$\text{Dose (mL/hr)} = \frac{700 \text{ U}}{100 \text{ mL}}$$

$$\text{Dose (mL/hr)} = 7 \text{ mL/hr}$$

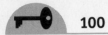

The Heparin Subcutaneous Formula

Heparin can also be ordered as an s.c. injection. In the order, the physician specifies the number of units of heparin that the patient should receive. You must calculate the dose to administer to the patient using the heparin subcutaneous formula.

The heparin subcutaneous formula should look familiar to you because it is the same formula used to calculate doses for other medication that you learned in Chapter 2.

Here's the formula:

$$\text{Dose} = \frac{\text{ordered}}{\text{on hand}} \times \text{quantity}$$

Let's say the order reads:

Heparin 5000 U s.c. daily

The label reads heparin 20,000 U/mL. Here's how to calculate the dose:

1. Insert values into the formula.

$$\text{Dose} = \frac{5000 \text{ U}}{20,000} \times 1 \text{ mL}$$

2. Calculate.

$$\text{Dose} = 0.25 \text{ U} \times 1 \text{ mL}$$
$$\text{Dose} = 0.25 \text{ mL}$$

Practice Drill 6.2—the Heparin Subcutaneous Formula

Calculate the following doses:

1. Medication order: heparin 5000 U s.c. daily
   Medication label: heparin 20,000 U/2 mL

   How many milliliters will be administered to the patient?

2. Medication order: heparin 4000 U s.c. daily
   Medication label: heparin 10,000 U/mL

   How many milliliters will be administered to the patient?

3. Medication order: heparin 2500 U s.c. daily
   Medication label: heparin 25,000 U/10 mL

   How many milliliters will be administered to the patient?

4. Medication order: heparin 2000 U s.c. daily
   Medication label: 20,000 U heparin/5 mL

   How many milliliters will be administered to the patient?

5. Medication order: heparin 7500 U s.c. daily
   Medication label: 20,000 U heparin/2 mL

   How many milliliters will be administered to the patient?

6. Medication order: heparin 8000 U s.c. daily
   Medication label: 20,000 U heparin/10 mL

   How many milliliters will be administered to the patient?

7. Medication order: heparin 6250 U/hr
   Medication label: 25,000 U heparin/4 mL

   How many milliliters will be administered to the patient?

8. Medication order: heparin 4000 U s.c. daily
   Medication label: 10,000 U heparin/5 mL

   How many milliliters will be administered to the patient?

9. Medication order: heparin 3000 U s.c. daily
   Medication label: 15,000 U heparin/5 mL

   How many milliliters will be administered to the patient?

10. Medication order: heparin 6000 U s.c. daily
    Medication label: 10,000 U heparin/5 mL

    How many milliliters will be administered to the patient?

Solutions to Practice Drill 6.2—the Heparin Subcutaneous Formula

1. $\text{Dose (mL/hr)} = \dfrac{5000 \text{ U}}{20,000 \text{ U}} \times 2 \text{ mL}$

   $\text{Dose (mL/hr)} = 0.25 \text{ U} \times 2 \text{ mL}$

   $\text{Dose (mL/hr)} = 0.5 \text{ mL}$

2. $\text{Dose (mL/hr)} = \dfrac{4000 \text{ U}}{10{,}000 \text{ U}} \times 1 \text{ mL}$

   $\text{Dose (mL/hr)} = 0.4 \text{ U} \times 1 \text{ mL}$

   $\text{Dose (mL/hr)} = 0.4 \text{ mL}$

3. $\text{Dose (mL/hr)} = \dfrac{2500 \text{ U}}{25{,}000 \text{ U}} \times 10 \text{ mL}$

   $\text{Dose (mL/hr)} = 0.1 \text{ U} \times 10 \text{ mL}$

   $\text{Dose (mL/hr)} = 1 \text{ mL}$

4. $\text{Dose (mL/hr)} = \dfrac{2000 \text{ U}}{20{,}000 \text{ U}} \times 5 \text{ mL}$

   $\text{Dose (mL/hr)} = 0.1 \text{ U} \times 5 \text{ mL}$

   $\text{Dose (mL/hr)} = 0.5 \text{ mL}$

5. $\text{Dose (mL/hr)} = \dfrac{7500 \text{ U}}{20{,}000 \text{ U}} \times 2 \text{ mL}$

   $\text{Dose (mL/hr)} = 0.375 \text{ U} \times 2 \text{ mL}$

   $\text{Dose (mL/hr)} = 0.75 \text{ mL}$

6. $\text{Dose (mL/hr)} = \dfrac{8000 \text{ U}}{20{,}000 \text{ U}} \times 10 \text{ mL}$

   $\text{Dose (mL/hr)} = 0.4 \text{ U} \times 10 \text{ mL}$

   $\text{Dose (mL/hr)} = 4 \text{ mL}$

7. $\text{Dose (mL/hr)} = \dfrac{6250 \text{ U}}{25{,}000 \text{ U}} \times 4 \text{ mL}$

   $\text{Dose (mL/hr)} = 0.25 \text{ U} \times 4 \text{ mL}$

   $\text{Dose (mL/hr)} = 1 \text{ mL}$

8. $\text{Dose (mL/hr)} = \dfrac{4000 \text{ U}}{10{,}000 \text{ U}} \times 5 \text{ mL}$

   $\text{Dose (mL/hr)} = 0.4 \text{ U} \times 5 \text{ mL}$

   $\text{Dose (mL/hr)} = 2 \text{ mL}$

9. Dose (mL/hr) = $\dfrac{3000 \text{ U}}{15{,}000 \text{ U}} \times 5$ mL

   Dose (mL/hr) = 0.2 U × 5 mL

   Dose (mL/hr) = 1 mL

10. Dose (mL/hr) = $\dfrac{6000 \text{ U}}{10{,}000 \text{ U}} \times 5$ mL

    Dose (mL/hr) = 0.6 U × 5 mL

    Dose (mL/hr) = 3 mL

CAUTION *Before administering heparin determine the number of units of heparin that the patient has received within the last 24 hours. If the total number of units including the next dose is greater than 40,000 units, then don't administer the next dose and notify the physician. Adult patients should not receive more than 40,000 units per 24 hour period.*

Summary

Heparin is an **anticoagulant** that is administered I.V. or s.c. and is measured in USP units (U). The prescribed dose of heparin is based on the partial thromboplastin time test, which determines the therapeutic level. Physicians order heparin as a number of units per hour for I.V. administration or a number of units for an s.c. injection.

Calculating the pump setting to administer heparin I.V. to the patient is a two-step process. First, calculate the number of units of heparin in 1 mL of I.V. fluid and then use this to calculate the number of milliliters of the I.V. fluid to administer to the patient per hour.

Calculate the dose for an s.c. injection by using the same method as is used to calculate medication that you learned in Chapter 2.

Quiz

1. The physician ordered heparin 500 U/hr. The medication label reads 20,000 U heparin in 200-mL normal saline. How many milliliters will be administered to the patient per hour?

a. 50 mL

b. 500 mL

c. 5 mL

d. 0.5 mL

2. The physician ordered heparin 800 U/hr. The medication label reads 25,000 U heparin in 250-mL D5W. How many milliliters will be administered to the patient per hour?

   a. 7.5 mL

   b. 7 mL

   c. 8 mL

   d. 8.5 mL

3. The physician ordered heparin 6000 U s.c. The medication label reads 10,000 U heparin/10 mL. How many milliliters will be administered to the patient?

   a. 5 mL

   b. 6 mL

   c. 6.5 mL

   d. 7 mL

4. The physician ordered heparin 20000 U/hr. The medication label reads 2000 U heparin in 20-mL normal saline. Two milliliters will be administered to the patient per hour.

   a. True

   b. False

5. The physician ordered heparin 5250 U s.c.. The medication label reads 15,000 U heparin/5 mL. How many milliliters will be administered to the patient per hour?

   a. 1.25 mL

   b. 1 mL

   c. 1.75 mL

   d. 2 mL

6. The physician ordered heparin 400 U/hr. The medication label reads 20,000 U heparin in 400-mL normal saline. How many milliliters will be administered to the patient per hour?

   a. 9 mL

   b. 8 mL

c. 7 mL

   d. 6 mL

7. The physician ordered heparin 100 U/hr. The medication label reads 20,000 U heparin in 2000 mL D5W. How many milliliters will be administered to the patient per hour?

   a. 1 mL

   b. 1.9 mL

   c. 0.9 mL

   d. 10 mL

8. The physician ordered heparin 4500 U s.c. The medication label reads 10,000 U heparin-5 mL. How many milliliters will be administered to the patient per hour?

   a. 2.25 mL

   b. 2.50 mL

   c. 2 mL

   d. 3 mL

9. The physician ordered heparin 600 U/hr. The medication label reads 25,000 U heparin in 500-mL normal saline. How many milliliters will be administered to the patient per hour?

   a. 0.2 mL

   b. 1.2 mL

   c. 0.12 mL

   d. 12 mL

10. The physician ordered heparin 800 U/hr. The medication label reads 10,000 U heparin in 250-mL D5W. How many milliliters will be administered to the patient per hour?

   a. 20 mL

   b. 2.1 mL

   c. 2 mL

   d. 21 mL

CHAPTER 7

Calculating Dopamine Dose

Dopamine is a neurotransmitter formed in the brain that affects movement, emotion, and perception. An imbalance or absence of dopamine can result in the patient having unnatural movement, irrational thoughts, and other signs and symptoms associated with Parkinson's disease, bipolar disorder, schizophrenia, and paranoia. Physicians prescribe dopamine to bring dopamine into balance and return the patient to normal movement, emotions, and perceptions. Dopamine is also frequently prescribed for kidney perfusion and for coronary conditions.

Calculating the proper dose of dopamine to administer to your patient is a little different from the way you calculate the dose of other medications because the prescribed dose is per kilogram and the medication on hand is a concentration. A concentration is a mixture of intravenous (I.V.) fluid that contains a specific amount of dopamine.

Before you calculate the dose for your patient, you must use the prescribed dose to calculate prescribed dose for your patient's weight and you also need to calculate the amount of dopamine in a milliliter of the concentration. You'll learn these calculations in this chapter.

Learning Objectives

➤ Calculating dopamine dose
➤ The dopamine dose calculation formula

Key Words

Bipolar disorder

Concentration

Dopamine

Neurotransmitter

Parkinson's disease

Calculating Dopamine Dose

There are several steps that you must perform to calculate the proper dose of **dopamine** to administer to your patient. Nearly all you used to calculate other medication throughout this book.

Dopamine is prescribed by weight similar to pediatric medication (see Chapter 5). The physician prescribes a dose per kilogram of the patient's weight, which means that you'll have to convert the patient's weight from pounds to kilograms in order to calculate the dose to administer to the patient.

Dopamine is administered intravenously using an infusion pump. The dose prescribed by the physician is for a minute infusion. The dose entered into I.V. infusion pumps is for an hour of infusion, which requires you to adjust the prescribed dose from a minute to an hour.

Dopamine comes premixed in an I.V. fluid from the pharmacy. You must calculate the **concentration** of dopamine in a milliliter of I.V. fluid, which is then used to calculate the dose of dopamine to administer to the patient.

Here's an example of a dopamine order:

Dopamine 3 mcg/kg . min

The Dopamine Dose Calculation Formula

There are three steps in calculating the dose of dopamine to administer to your patient. The first step is to convert your patient's weight to kilograms, if your patient's weight is recorded in pounds. You'll recall from Chapter 5 that 1 kg = 2.2 lb.

Convert your patient's weight from pounds to kilograms by dividing your patient's weight in pounds by 2.2.

The second step is to calculate the concentration of dopamine in 1 mL of I.V. fluid. This is similar to calculating the concentration of heparin that you learned to do in Chapter 6. The I.V. solution container specifies the total amount of milliliters and the total amount of dopamine in the container. You need to calculate the concentration of dopamine in 1 mL of I.V. fluid. You do this by dividing the amount of dopamine in the I.V. container by the amount of I.V. fluid. The result is the concentration—the number of milligrams of dopamine in 1 mL of I.V. fluid.

The third step is to calculate the dose to administer to your patient.

Here's the dopamine formula:

1. Convert the patient's weight from pounds to kilograms.

$$\text{Weight (kg)} = \frac{\text{weight (lb)}}{2.2}$$

2. Calculate the concentration of dopamine that is delivered from the pharmacy

$$\text{Concentration} = \frac{\text{on hand (mg)}}{\text{on hand (mL)}}$$

3. Calculate the dose to administer to your patient. Remember that the prescribed dose is for 1 minute and that the infusion pump is set for 1 hour. Therefore, you must multiply by 60 minutes.

$$\text{Dose (mL/hr)} = \frac{\text{ordered (mg)} \times \text{weight (kg)} \times 60 \text{ minute}}{\text{concentration}}$$

HINT *The prescribed dose of dopamine might be in micrograms (mcg) and the I.V. solution delivered by the pharmacy has dopamine in milligrams (mg). Therefore you must convert the amount of dopamine in the I.V. bag from milligrams to micrograms before calculating the dose to administer to your patients. You convert milligrams to micrograms by multiplying the milligrams by 1000 (see Chapter 2 Converting Metric Units).*

CALCULATING USING THE FORMULA

Say that the physician wrote the following prescription for your patient who weighs 165 lb:

Dopamine 3 mcg/kg·min

The pharmacy delivered an I.V.–labeled dopamine 400 mg in 250 D5W. Here's how to calculate the dose to administer to your patient:

1. Convert your patient's weight from pounds to kilograms.

$$75 \text{ kg} = \frac{165 \text{ lb}}{2.2 \text{ lb}}$$

2. Calculate the dopamine concentration in the I.V. fluid.

$$400,000 \text{ mcg} = 400 \text{ mg} \times 1000$$
$$1600 \text{ mcg} = \frac{400,000}{250 \text{ mL}}$$

3. Calculate the dose.

$$\text{Dose (mL/hr)} = \frac{3 \text{ mcg} \times 75 \text{ kg} \times 60 \text{ minute}}{1600 \text{ mcg}}$$
$$\text{Dose (mL/hr)} = \frac{225 \text{ mcg} \times 60 \text{ minute}}{1600 \text{ mcg}}$$
$$\text{Dose (mL/hr)} = \frac{13,500 \text{ mcg}}{1600 \text{ mcg}}$$
$$\text{Dose (mL/hr)} = 8.437 = 8 \text{ mL/hr}$$

Practice Drill 7.1—the Dopamine Dose Calculation Formula

Calculate the following doses:

1. Medication order: dopamine 5 mcg/kg·min for a patient that weighs 178 lb
    Medication label: dopamine 800 mg in 500 D5W

    How many milliliters will be administered to the patient per hour?

2. Medication order: dopamine 7 mcg/kg·min for a patient that weighs 190 lb
    Medication label: dopamine 800 mg in 500 D5W

    How many milliliters will be administered to the patient per hour?

3. Medication order: dopamine 8 mcg/kg·min for a patient that weighs 165 lb

   Medication label: dopamine 400 mg in 250 D5W

   How many milliliters will be administered to the patient per hour?

4. Medication order: dopamine 4 mcg/kg·min for a patient that weighs 184 lb

   Medication label: dopamine 400 mg in 250 D5W

   How many milliliters will be administered to the patient per hour?

5. Medication order: dopamine 7 mcg/kg·min for a patient that weighs 155 lb

   Medication label: dopamine 800 mg in 500 D5W

   How many milliliters will be administered to the patient per hour?

6. Medication order: dopamine 5 mcg/kg·min for a patient that weighs 175 lb

   Medication label: dopamine 400 mg in 250 D5W

   How many milliliters will be administered to the patient per hour?

7. Medication order: dopamine 7 mcg/kg·min for a patient that weighs 190 lb

   Medication label: dopamine 800 mg in 500 D5W

   How many milliliters will be administered to the patient per hour?

8. Medication order: dopamine 5 mcg/kg·min for a patient that weighs 185 lb

   Medication label: dopamine 400 mg in 250 D5W

   How many milliliters will be administered to the patient per hour?

9. Medication order: dopamine 3 mcg/kg·min for a patient that weighs 172 lb

   Medication label: dopamine 400 mg in 250 D5W

   How many milliliters will be administered to the patient per hour?

10. Medication order: dopamine 5 mcg/kg·min for a patient that weighs 200 lb

    Medication label: dopamine 800 mg in 500 D5W

    How many milliliters will be administered to the patient per hour?

Solutions to Practice Drill 7.1—the Dopamine Dose Calculation Formula

1. $80.909 \text{ kg} = \dfrac{178 \text{ lb}}{2.2 \text{ lb}}$

$800,000 \text{ mcg} = 800 \text{ mg} \times 1000$

$1600 \text{ mcg} = \dfrac{800,000 \text{ mcg}}{500 \text{ mL}}$

$\text{Dose (mL/hr)} = \dfrac{5 \text{ mcg} \times 80.909 \text{ kg} \times 60 \text{ minutes}}{1600 \text{ mcg}}$

$\text{Dose (mL/hr)} = \dfrac{404.545 \text{ mcg} \times 60 \text{ minutes}}{1600 \text{ mcg}}$

$\text{Dose (mL/hr)} = \dfrac{24,272.7 \text{ mcg}}{1600 \text{ mcg}}$

$\text{Dose (mL/hr)} = 15.17 = 15 \text{ mL/hr}$

2. $86.363 \text{ kg} = \dfrac{190 \text{ lb}}{2.2 \text{ lb}}$

$800,000 \text{ mcg} = 800 \text{ mg} \times 1000$

$1600 \text{ mcg} = \dfrac{800,000 \text{ mcg}}{500 \text{ mL}}$

$\text{Dose (mL/hr)} = \dfrac{7 \text{ mcg} \times 86.363 \text{ kg} \times 60 \text{ minutes}}{1600 \text{ mcg}}$

$\text{Dose (mL/hr)} = \dfrac{604.54 \text{ mcg} \times 60 \text{ minutes}}{1600 \text{ mcg}}$

$\text{Dose (mL/hr)} = \dfrac{36,272.5}{1600 \text{ mcg}}$

$\text{Dose (mL/hr)} = 22.67 = 23 \text{ mL/hr}$

3. $$75 \text{ kg} = \frac{165 \text{ lb}}{2.2 \text{ lb}}$$

$$400,000 \text{ mcg} = 400 \text{ mg} \times 1000$$

$$1600 \text{ mcg} = \frac{400,000 \text{ mcg}}{250 \text{ mL}}$$

$$\text{Dose (mL/hr)} = \frac{8 \text{ mcg} \times 75 \text{ kg} \times 60 \text{ minutes}}{1600 \text{ mcg}}$$

$$\text{Dose (mL/hr)} = \frac{600 \text{ mcg} \times 60 \text{ minutes}}{1600 \text{ mcg}}$$

$$\text{Dose (mL/hr)} = \frac{36,000 \text{ mcg}}{1600 \text{ mcg}}$$

$$\text{Dose (mL/hr)} = 22.5 = 23 \text{ mL/hr}$$

4. $$83.636 \text{ kg} = \frac{184 \text{ lb}}{2.2 \text{ lb}}$$

$$400,000 \text{ mcg} = 400 \text{ mg} \times 1000$$

$$1600 \text{ mcg} = \frac{400,000 \text{ mcg}}{250 \text{ mL}}$$

$$\text{Dose (mL/hr)} = \frac{4 \text{ mcg} \times 83.636 \text{ kg} \times 60 \text{ minutes}}{1600 \text{ mcg}}$$

$$\text{Dose (mL/hr)} = \frac{334.544 \text{ mcg} \times 60 \text{ minutes}}{1600 \text{ mcg}}$$

$$\text{Dose (mL/hr)} = \frac{20,072.64 \text{ mcg}}{1600 \text{ mcg}}$$

$$\text{Dose (mL/hr)} = 12.545 = 13 \text{ mL/hr}$$

5. $\quad 70.454 \text{ kg} = \dfrac{155 \text{ lb}}{2.2 \text{ lb}}$

$800,000 \text{ mcg} = 800 \text{ mg} \times 1000$

$1600 \text{ mcg} = \dfrac{800,000 \text{ mcg}}{500 \text{ mL}}$

$\text{Dose (mL/hr)} = \dfrac{7 \text{ mcg} \times 70.454 \text{ kg} \times 60 \text{ minutes}}{1600 \text{ mcg}}$

$\text{Dose (mL/hr)} = \dfrac{493.178 \text{ mcg} \times 60 \text{ minutes}}{1600 \text{ mcg}}$

$\text{Dose (mL/hr)} = \dfrac{29,590.68 \text{ mcg}}{1600 \text{ mcg}}$

$\text{Dose (mL/hr)} = 18.494 = 19 \text{ mL/hr}$

6. $\quad 79.545 \text{ kg} = \dfrac{175 \text{ lb}}{2.2 \text{ lb}}$

$400,000 \text{ mcg} = 400 \text{ mg} \times 1000$

$1600 \text{ mcg} = \dfrac{400,000 \text{ mcg}}{250 \text{ mL}}$

$\text{Dose (mL/hr)} = \dfrac{5 \text{ mcg} \times 79.545 \text{ kg} \times 60 \text{ minutes}}{1600 \text{ mcg}}$

$\text{Dose (mL/hr)} = \dfrac{397.725 \text{ mcg} \times 60 \text{ minutes}}{1600 \text{ mcg}}$

$\text{Dose (mL/hr)} = \dfrac{23,863.5 \text{ mcg}}{1600 \text{ mcg}}$

$\text{Dose (mL/hr)} = 14.914 = 15 \text{ mL/hr}$

7. $86.363 \text{ kg} = \dfrac{190 \text{ lb}}{2.2 \text{ lb}}$

$800{,}000 \text{ mcg} = 800 \text{ mg} \times 1000$

$1600 \text{ mcg} = \dfrac{800{,}000 \text{ mcg}}{500 \text{ mL}}$

$\text{Dose (mL/hr)} = \dfrac{7 \text{ mcg} \times 86.363 \text{ kg} \times 60 \text{ minutes}}{1600 \text{ mcg}}$

$\text{Dose (mL/hr)} = \dfrac{604.541 \text{ mcg} \times 60 \text{ minutes}}{1600 \text{ mcg}}$

$\text{Dose (mL/hr)} = \dfrac{36{,}272.46 \text{ mcg}}{1600 \text{ mcg}}$

$\text{Dose (mL/hr)} = 22.67 = 23 \text{ mL/hr}$

8. $84.09 \text{ kg} = \dfrac{185 \text{ lb}}{2.2 \text{ lb}}$

$400{,}000 \text{ mcg} = 400 \text{ mg} \times 1000$

$1600 \text{ mcg} = \dfrac{400{,}000 \text{ mcg}}{250 \text{ mL}}$

$\text{Dose (mL/hr)} = \dfrac{5 \text{ mcg} \times 84.09 \text{ kg} \times 60 \text{ minutes}}{1600 \text{ mcg}}$

$\text{Dose (mL/hr)} = \dfrac{420.45 \text{ mcg} \times 60 \text{ minutes}}{1600 \text{ mcg}}$

$\text{Dose (mL/hr)} = \dfrac{25{,}227 \text{ mcg}}{1600 \text{ mcg}}$

$\text{Dose (mL/hr)} = 15.766 = 16 \text{ mL/hr}$

9. $$78.181 \text{ kg} = \frac{172 \text{ lb}}{2.2 \text{ lb}}$$

$$400{,}000 \text{ mcg} = 400 \text{ mg} \times 1000$$

$$1600 \text{ mcg} = \frac{400{,}000 \text{ mcg}}{250 \text{ mL}}$$

$$\text{Dose (mL/hr)} = \frac{3 \text{ mcg} \times 78.181 \text{ kg} \times 60 \text{ minutes}}{1600 \text{ mcg}}$$

$$\text{Dose (mL/hr)} = \frac{234.543 \text{ mcg} \times 60 \text{ minutes}}{1600 \text{ mcg}}$$

$$\text{Dose (mL/hr)} = \frac{14{,}072.58 \text{ mcg}}{1600 \text{ mcg}}$$

$$\text{Dose (mL/hr)} = 8.795 = 9 \text{ mL/hr}$$

10. $$90.909 \text{ kg} = \frac{200 \text{ lb}}{2.2 \text{ lb}}$$

$$800{,}000 \text{ mcg} = 800 \text{ mg} \times 1000$$

$$1600 \text{ mcg} = \frac{800{,}000 \text{ mcg}}{500 \text{ mL}}$$

$$\text{Dose (mL/hr)} = \frac{5 \text{ mcg} \times 90.909 \text{ kg} \times 60 \text{ minutes}}{1600 \text{ mcg}}$$

$$\text{Dose (mL/hr)} = \frac{454.545 \text{ mcg} \times 60 \text{ minutes}}{1600 \text{ mcg}}$$

$$\text{Dose (mL/hr)} = \frac{27{,}272.7 \text{ mcg}}{1600 \text{ mcg}}$$

$$\text{Dose (mL/hr)} = 17.045 = 17 \text{ mL/hr}$$

Summary

Dopamine is a **neurotransmitter** formed in the brain that affects movement, emotion, and perception. A decrease in dopamine causes symptoms associated with **Parkinson's disease** and some psychotic conditions. It is also used for renal perfusion and cardiac conditions.

Dopamine is prescribed by a dose per kilogram of the patient's weight and infused for 1 minute. The patient's weight must be converted from pounds to kilogram and then you must calculate the dose to be infused for an hour.

The pharmacy delivers dopamine in a concentration of a volume of I.V. fluid. You must calculate the amount of dopamine in a milliliter of I.V. fluid in order to calculate the dose that you are to administer to your patient.

Quiz

1. The physician ordered dopamine 8 mcg/kg·min for a patient that weighs 220 lb. The pharmacy delivers dopamine 400 mg in 250 D5W. How many milliliters per hour will you set the infusion pump?

    a.   30 mL

    b.   29.5 mL

    c.   31 mL

    d.   29 mL

2. The physician ordered dopamine 3 mcg/kg·min for a patient that weighs 132 lb. The pharmacy delivers dopamine 400 mg in 250 D5W. How many milliliters per hour will you set the infusion pump?

    a.   6.5 mL

    b.   6.25 mL

    c.   6 mL

    d.   6.75 mL

3. The physician ordered dopamine 6 mcg/kg·min for a patient that weighs 154 lb. The pharmacy delivers dopamine 800 mg in 500 D5W. How many milliliters per hour will you set the infusion pump?

    a.   15 mL

    b.   16 mL

    c.   14 mL

    d.   17 mL

4. The physician ordered dopamine 5 mcg/kg·min for a patient that weighs 187 lb. The pharmacy delivers dopamine 400 mg in 250 D5W. The infusion pump should be set to 16 mL per hour.

   a. True

   b. False

5. The physician ordered dopamine 3 mcg/kg·min for a patient that weighs 131 lb. The pharmacy delivers dopamine 800 mg in 500 D5W. How many milliliters per hour will you set the infusion pump?

   a. 7 mL

   b. 6 mL

   c. 6.7 mL

   d. 6.8 mL

6. The physician ordered dopamine 7 mcg/kg·min for a patient that weighs 240 lb. The pharmacy delivers dopamine 400 mg in 250 D5W. How many milliliters per hour will you set the infusion pump?

   a. 28 mL

   b. 29 mL

   c. 28.6 mL

   d. 28.63 mL

7. The physician ordered dopamine 3 mcg/kg·min for a patient that weighs 180 lb. The pharmacy delivers dopamine 400 mg in 250 D5W. How many milliliters per hour will you set the infusion pump?

   a. 10 mL

   b. 9.2 mL

   c. 9 mL

   d. 9.5 mL

8. The physician ordered dopamine 4 mcg/kg·min for a patient that weighs 195 lb. The pharmacy delivers dopamine 800 mg in 500 D5W. How many milliliters per hour will you set the infusion pump?

   a. 13 mL

   b. 14 mL

   c. 13.7 mL

   d. 13.29 mL

9. The physician ordered dopamine 5 mcg/kg·min for a patient that weighs 171 lb. The pharmacy delivers dopamine 800 mg in 500 D5W. How many milliliters per hour will you set the infusion pump?

   a.　1.5 mL

   b.　14.6 mL

   c.　14 mL

   d.　15 mL

10. The physician ordered dopamine 5 mcg/kg·min for a patient that weighs 215 lb. The pharmacy delivers dopamine 400 mg in 250 D5W. How many milliliters per hour will you set the infusion pump?

    a.　18.715 mL

    b.　18.71 mL

    c.　18.3 mL

    d.　18 mL

CHAPTER 8

Calculating Dose for Children Using Body Surface Area

Weight-based dose calculations, which you learned in Chapter 5, references one measurement of a child—weight—to calculate the proper dose. Some physicians prefer to use the child's body surface area (BSA) rather than weight as the basis for calculating the dose.

Body surface area reflects both the child's weight and height and is considered to be the most accurate way to calculate a dose for a child because it considers two measurement of a child.

In this chapter you'll learn how to calculate the proper dose of medication for your young patient by using the child's BSA.

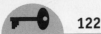

Learning Objectives

➤ What is body surface area?

➤ Why calculate the surface area?

➤ Calculating the body surface area

➤ The BSA child dose calculation formula

Key Words	
Adult dose	Metabolic mass
Body surface area	Metabolism
BSA	Square meters
Du Bois & Du Bois formula	Surface area
	West nomogram

What Is Body Surface Area?

Remember back in grammar school math when the teacher asked how many 1-ft square tiles are needed to cover the area of the kitchen floor. The teacher was really asking you to calculate the **surface area** of the kitchen floor.

Think of the surface area of a person as being similar to the surface area of the kitchen floor—with some obvious exceptions. The person's body has a relatively irregular shape and has more than two dimensions. You can't simply take a rule and measure every foot of the body like you can the kitchen floor.

However, aside from these differences, there are similarities between the surface area of the kitchen floor and the surface area of a person's body. Both have an area that covers it (i.e., the floor and the body) called the surface area. And the surface area can be calculated using a mathematical formula, although a different formula is used to calculate the surface area of the body than is used to calculate the surface area of the kitchen floor.

WHY CALCULATE THE SURFACE AREA?

After a medication is administered and absorbed into the body, the body breaks down the medication into components, which is referred to as metabolizing the medication. The components enter the blood stream where they are distributed throughout the body and eventually excreted.

The rate at which the medication is metabolized influences the dose that is prescribed to the patient. The goal is for the physician to prescribe a dose that achieves a therapeutic level without resulting in an overdose.

If the dose is too high for **metabolism**, then this could lead to an overdose because a second dose is administered before the first dose is fully metabolized. If the dose is too low for the metabolism, then the medication could be excreted before the next dose is administered resulting is the medication never reaching a therapeutic level in the blood.

The patient's **metabolic mass** influences the rate at which the medication is metabolized. While the patient's weight is a good indicator of a patient's metabolic mass, the patient's **body surface area** is even a better indicator of metabolic mass.

Therefore, some physicians prefer to use body surface area rather than weight to prescribe medication. This is especially true when highly sensitive medication such as chemotherapy is being prescribed.

Calculating the Body Surface Area

Unfortunately, the formula for calculating the body surface area is more complicated that the formula used to calculate how many 1-ft tiles are needed to cover the kitchen floor. There are several formulas that can be used to calculate the **BSA**. The **Du Bois & Du Bois formula** is commonly used. Here it is:

$$BSA = (71.84 \times \text{weight (kg)}^{0.425} \times \text{height (cm)}^{0.725})/10,000$$

But don't sweat the math because the math to calculate the body surface area is done for you if you use **West nomogram** (Figure 8.1). A nomogram is a chart that shows the relationship among values. The West nomogram shows the relationship among the patient's height, weight, and body surface area.

The West nomogram is divided into three sets of numbers. The first set is height in inches, the second set is body surface, and the third set is weight in pounds. These sets are lined up together based on the Du Bois & Du Bois formula.

Here's how to use the West nomogram to calculate the patient's body surface area:

1. Measure the patient's height in centimeters or inches.
2. Weight the patient in kilogram or pounds.

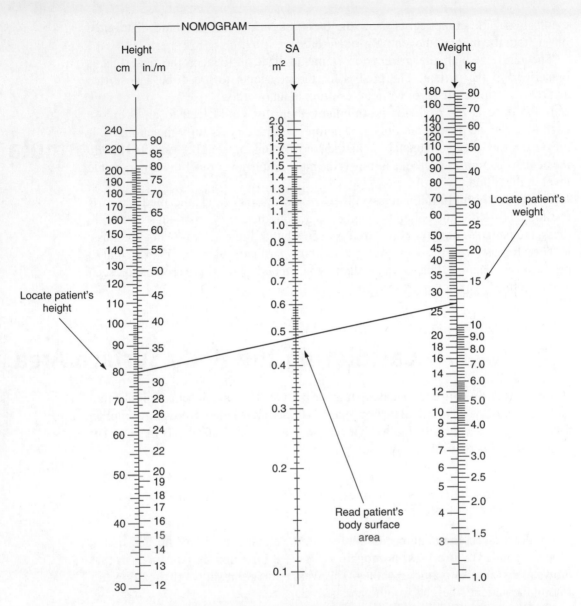

Figure 8.1 Draw a line from the patient's height to the patient's weight on the West nomogram and the line intersects the patient's body surface. (*Modified from data of E. Boyd by C.D. West; from Behrman, R.E., Kliegman, R.M., & Jenson, H.B. (eds.). (2000). Nelson Textbook of Pediatrics (16th ed.). Philadelphia: W.B. Saunders.*)

3. Draw a line from the patient's height in the height set of numbers on the West nomogram to the patient's weight in the weight set of numbers.

4. The line intersects a number on the body surface set of numbers. This is the patient's body surface area in **square meters** (m²).

The BSA Child Dose Calculation Formula

You probably realize that an **adult dose** of a medication is too much of a dose to administer to a child because the child is much smaller than the adult. Then what is the proper dose for a child?

You determine the proper dose for a child by using the following formula that uses both the child's body surface area and the adult dose:

$$\text{Child dose} = \frac{\text{body surface area (m}^2)}{1.73 \text{ m}^2} \times \text{adult dose}$$

CALCULATING USING THE FORMULA

Let's say that the child is 32 in tall and weighs 25 lb. The physician orders Demerol with the adult dose of 100 mg. Your job is to calculate the dose to administer to the child.

1. Determine the child's body surface area. You do this by drawing a line from 32 in in the height set of number to 25 lb in the weight set of numbers on the West nomogram. In doing so, you'll notice that the line intersects 0.50 m² in the body surface set of numbers. This is the child's body surface area.

2. Enter the body surface area and the adult dose into the formula.

$$\text{Child dose} = \frac{0.5 \text{ m}^2}{1.73 \text{ m}^2} \times 100 \text{ mg}$$

3. Divide the child's body surface area by 1.73 m².

$$\text{Child dose} = 0.289 \times 100 \text{ mg}$$

4. Multiply the adult dose by 0.289 to arrive at the child's dose.

$$\text{Child dose} = 28.9 \text{ mg}$$

HINT *Think of 0.289 or whatever value is calculated as the percentage of the adult dose. In this example, the child's dose based on this child's body surface area is 28.9% of the adult dose. Remember that this percentage changes based on the child's body surface.*

Practice Drill 8.1—the BSA Child Dose Calculation Formula

Calculate the following doses:

1. The child is 85 cm tall and weighs 25 lb and the adult dose of Capoten is 6.25 mg.

   How many milligrams will be administered to your patient?

2. The child is 42 in tall and weighs 40 lb and the adult dose of Decadron is 3 mg.

   How many milligrams will be administered to your patient?

3. The child is 44 in tall and weighs 50 lb and the adult dose of Cephalexin is 125 mg.

   How many milligrams will be administered to your patient?

4. The child is 70 cm tall and weighs 9 kg and the adult dose of Zovirax is 25 mg.

   How many milligrams will be administered to your patient?

5. The child is 45 cm in tall and weighs 3 kg and the adult dose of Celocin is 125 mg.

   How many milligrams will be administered to your patient?

6. The child is 21 in tall and weighs 10 lb and the adult dose of Zofran is 2000 mcg.

   How many milligrams will be administered to your patient?

7. The child is 75 in tall and weighs 25 lb and the adult dose of Ampicillin is 100 mg.

   How many milligrams will be administered to your patient?

8. The child is 41 in tall and weighs 60 lb and the adult dose of Lithostat is 250 mg.

   How many milligrams will be administered to your patient?

9. The child is 105 cm tall and weighs 25 kg and the adult dose of Benylin is 50 mg.

   How many milligrams will be administered to your patient?

10. The child is 80 cm tall and weighs 25 lb and the adult dose of Amoxicillin is 125 mg.

   How many milligrams will be administered to your patient?

Solutions to Practice Drill 8.1—the BSA Child Dose Calculation Formula

1. $1.8 \text{ mg} = \dfrac{0.5 \text{ m}^2}{1.73 \text{ m}^2} \times 6.25 \text{ mg}$

2. $1.3 \text{ mg} - \dfrac{0.75 \text{ m}^2}{1.73 \text{ m}^2} \times 3 \text{ mg}$

3. $61.4 \text{ mg} = \dfrac{0.85 \text{ m}^2}{1.73 \text{ m}^2} \times 125 \text{ mg}$

4. $5.8 \text{ mg} = \dfrac{0.4 \text{ m}^2}{1.73 \text{ m}^2} \times 25 \text{ mg}$

5. $13 \text{ mg} = \dfrac{0.18 \text{ m}^2}{1.73 \text{ m}^2} \times 125 \text{ mg}$

6. $289 \text{ mcg} = \dfrac{0.25 \text{ m}^2}{1.73 \text{ m}^2} \times 2000 \text{ mcg}$

7. $27.2 \text{ mg} = \dfrac{0.47 \text{ m}^2}{1.73 \text{ m}^2} \times 100 \text{ mg}$

8. $122.8 \text{ mg} = \dfrac{0.85 \text{ m}^2}{1.73 \text{ m}^2} \times 250 \text{ mg}$

9. $24 \text{ mg} = \dfrac{0.83 \text{ m}^2}{1.73 \text{ m}^2} \times 50 \text{ mg}$

10. $35.4 \text{ mg} = \dfrac{0.49 \text{ m}^2}{1.73 \text{ m}^2} \times 125 \text{ mg}$

Summary

Some physicians prefer to use the child's body surface area rather than the child's weight as the basis for calculating the dose of a medication. The body surface area method is considered the most accurate way to calculate a dose.

The Du Bois & Du Bois formula is used to calculate the body surface area; however the West nomogram is used rather than the Du Bois & Du Bois formula. The West nomogram is a series of three sets of numbers: height, surface area, and weight.

You use the West nomogram by drawing a line from the child's height to the child's weight on the West nomogram. The line intersects the body surface area. The West nomogram displays inches and centimeters and pounds and kilograms.

The body surface area in square meters is used in a formula to calculate the child's dose based on the child's body surface area and the adult's dose for the medication.

Quiz

1. The adult dose ordered is Tegopen 125 mg for a patient who is 70 cm tall and weighs 20 lb. What dose would you administer to the patient?

    a. 32.5 mg

    b. 33.5 mg

    c. 30.1 mg

    d. 31.2 mg

2. The adult dose ordered is Ampicillin 100 mg for a patient who is 45 cm tall and weighs 7 lb. What dose would you administer to the patient?

    a. 10 mg

    b. 12.5 mg

    c. 11.6 mg

    d. 11 mg

3. The adult dose ordered is Cefotan 50 mg for a patient who is 30 in tall and weighs 25 lb. What dose would you administer to the patient?

    a. 13.8 mg

    b. 14.5 mg

    c. 13.7 mg

    d. 14 mg

4. The adult dose ordered is Ketzol 25 mg for a patient who is 36 in tall and weighs 15 kg. What dose would you administer to the patient?

   a. 8.7 mg

   b. 8 mg

   c. 8.5 mg

   d. 7.8 mg

5. The adult dose ordered is Erythrocin 50 mg for a patient who is 48 in tall and weighs 70 lb. What dose would you administer to the patient?

   a. 31.8 mg

   b. 28 mg

   c. 30 mg

   d. 29.8 mg

6. The adult dose ordered is Tetracycline 250 mg for a patient who is 43 in tall and weighs 25 kg. What dose would you administer to the patient?

   a. 96.1 mg

   b. 86.7 mg

   c. 84.1 mg

   d. 90.2 mg

7. The adult dose ordered is Trovan 100 mg for a patient who is 38 in tall and weighs 45 lb. What dose would you administer to the patient?

   a. 42 mg

   b. 42.1 mg

   c. 46.2 mg

   d. 42.3 mg

8. The adult dose ordered is Bactrim 30 mg for a patient who is 86 cm tall and weighs 30 lb. What dose would you administer to the patient?

   a. 10.4 mg

   b. 9.6 mg

   c. 9 mg

   d. 11.1 mg

9. The adult dose ordered is Sporanox 200 mg for a patient who is 60 cm tall and weighs 7 kg. What dose would you administer to the patient?

a. 36 mg

    b. 37.1 mg

    c. 36.9 mg

    d. 40.5 mg

10. The adult dose ordered is Flagyl 500 mg for a patient who is 70 cm tall and weighs 9 kg. What dose would you administer to the patient?

    a. 131.1 mg

    b. 128.7 mg

    c. 127.1 mg.

    d. 130 mg

CHAPTER 9

Enteral Tube Feeding

Patients who have a cardiovascular accident (CVA), tracheoesophageal fistula, esophageal atresia, or other conditions that affect swallowing are at risk for aspiration pneumonia and malnutrition. Physicians take the preemptive strategy of placing the patient on enteral tube feeding, which greatly reduces the risk for aspiration and assures that nutrients reach the stomach.

Enteral tube feedings usually come in full strength; however, the physician typically orders enteral tube feedings at less than full strength. This requires you to dilute the enteral tube feeding before it is administered to your patient.

In this chapter you'll learn how to calculate the fraction or percentage of dilution that must be applied to the full concentration of the enteral tube feeding.

Learning Objectives

➤ What is enteral tube feeding?

➤ Enteral tube feeding formula

➤ Enteral tube feeding formula by caloric intake

Key Words

Calories per ounce	Malnutrition
Concentration volume	Nasogastric feeding tube
Dilution factor	NG tube
Enteral tube	PEG tube
Enteral tube feeding concentration	Percutaneous endoscopic gastrostomy
Gastric feeding tube	Total volume

What Is Enteral Tube Feeding?

There are a number of conditions that can temporarily or permanently interfere with a patient's ability to swallow, placing the patient at risk for **malnutrition** and depletion of fat and muscle. In order to reduce this risk, the patient's physician orders the insertion of a feeding tube and **enteral tube** feeding.

There are two types of feeding tubes:

- Nasogastric feeding tube: The **nasogastric feeding tube** is commonly called an **NG tube** and is used for short-term enteral tube feedings. The NG tube passes through the patient's nares, then the esophagus, and into the stomach. Nutrients flow through the NG tube and go directly into the stomach without touching or affecting the esophagus.

- Gastric feeding tube: The **gastric feeding tube** is commonly called the **percutaneous endoscopic gastrostomy (PEG)** tube. The PEG tube is surgically placed through the abdominal wall and into the stomach. The PEG tube is held in place by either a balloon tip or by a retention dome. PEG tubes are replaced about every 6 months.

ENTERAL TUBE FEEDING CONCENTRATION

Imagine having a bottle of 100% orange juice. You can drink an 8-oz glass without having any uncomfortable feeling because you can tolerate 100% orange juice. However, someone else may not tolerate it as well, but does not have adverse effects if the 8-oz glass has 50% orange juice and 50% water. The problem is that the bottle contains 100% orange juice. This means that the orange juice must be diluted before being ingested.

This is similar in concept with enteral tube feedings except the feedings aren't orange juice. Depending on the patient's needs, the physician may order a special blend of nutrients that is prepared by the pharmacy, which meets the patient's requirements. Other times, the physician may order enteral tube feedings that are prepackaged, which may need to be diluted before being administered to the patient. You must calculate the dilution and prepare the enteral tube feeding.

Enteral Tube Feeding Formula

The physician will prescribe the strength of the prepackaged enteral food feeding that is to be administered to the patient. Prepackage enteral food feeding is 100% and the strength ordered by the physician is less than 100%.

The strength of the prepackaged enteral food feeding is reduced by diluting it with water. The enteral tube feeding formula determines the amount of water needed to dilute the prepackaged enteral food feeding to meet the strength ordered by the physician.

Before looking at the formula, it is important to understand these terms:

Concentration volume: This is the volume of the prepackaged enteral tube feeding, which is printed on the prepackage container.

Dilution factor: This is the strength specified by the physician's order and is given as a fraction or a percentage.

Total volume: This is the **total volume** of the enteral tube feeding after it has been diluted, which is the **concentration volume** and the added water.

Water to add: This is the amount of water you need to add to the prepackaged enteral food feeding to reach the total volume.

Calculating the amount of water to add to the prepackaged enteral food feeding is a two-step process.

1. Total volume = concentration volume/dilution factor
2. Water to add = total volume − concentration volume

CALCULATING USING THE ENTERAL TUBE FEEDING FORMULA

Let's say that the physician ordered the patient to receive enteral food feeding of Jevity at 1/2 strength via a PEG tube at 80 mL/hr. You have on hand a 240-mL can of Jevity at 100% strength. How much water is needed to dilute the can of Jevity?

1. 480 mL = 240 mL/0.50
2. 240 mL = 480 mL – 240 mL

Practice Drill 9.1—the Enteral Tube Feeding Formula

Calculate the following enteral tube feedings:

1. The physician ordered 100 cc of 1/4 strength Sustacal via a PEG tube. On hand is a 240-cc can of Sustacal, which is at full strength. How much water is needed to dilute Sustacal?

2. The physician ordered 160 cc of 3/4 strength Enrich via a PEG tube. On hand is a 240-cc can of Enrich, which is at full strength. How much water is needed to dilute Enrich?

3. The physician ordered 280 cc of 1/2 strength Jevity via an NG tube. On hand is a 150-cc can of Jevity, which is at full strength. How much water is needed to dilute Jevity?

4. The physician ordered 240 cc of 3/4 strength Jevity via an NG tube. On hand is a 12-oz can of Jevity, which is at full strength. How much water is needed to dilute Jevity?

5. The physician ordered 80 cc of 1/4 strength Enrich via a PEG tube. On hand is a 240-mL can of Enrich, which is at full strength. How much water is needed to dilute Enrich?

6. The physician ordered 260 cc of 1/5 strength Sustacal via a PEG tube. On hand is a 300-cc can of Sustacal, which is at full strength. How much water is needed to dilute Sustacal?

7. The physician ordered 280 cc of 1/3 strength Jevity via an NG tube. On hand is a 350-cc can of Jevity, which is at 100% strength. How much water is needed to dilute Jevity?

8. The physician ordered 180 cc of 3/5 strength Enrich via a PEG tube. On hand is a 480-mL can of Enrich, which is at full strength. How much water is needed to dilute Enrich?

9. The physician ordered 140 cc of 2/5 strength Sustacal via a PEG tube. On hand is a 360-cc can of Sustacal, which is at full strength. How much water is needed to dilute Sustacal?

10. The physician ordered 220 cc of 4/5 strength Enrich via an NG tube. On hand is a 12-oz can of Enrich, which is at 100% strength. How much water is needed to dilute Enrich?

Solutions to Practice Drill 9.1—the Enteral Tube Feeding Formula

1. 960 mL = 240 mL/0.25
   720 mL = 960 mL − 240 mL

2. 320 mL = 240 mL/0.75
   80 mL = 320 mL − 240 mL

3. 300 mL = 150 mL/0.5
   150 mL = 300 mL − 150 mL

4. 360 mL − 30 mL × 12 oz
   480 mL = 360 mL/0.75
   120 mL = 480 mL − 360 mL

5. 960 mL = 240 mL/0.25
   720 mL = 960 mL − 240 mL

6. 1500 mL = 300 mL/0.2
   1200 mL = 1500 mL − 300 mL

7. 1051 mL = 350 mL/0.333
   701 mL = 1051 mL − 350 mL

8. 800 mL = 480 mL/0.6
   320 mL = 800 mL − 480 mL

9. 900 mL = 360 mL/0.4
   540 mL = 900 mL − 360 mL

10. 360 mL = 30 mL × 12 oz
    450 mL = 360 mL/0.8
    90 mL = 450 mL − 360 mL

HINT *Convert a fraction to a decimal by dividing the numerator (top number) by the denominator (bottom number). For example, 2/5 is converted by dividing 2 by 5. The remainder is the decimal equivalent, which is 0.40.*

Convert a percentage to a decimal by dividing the percentage by 100. For example, 80%/100 = 0.80.

Enteral Tube Feeding Formula by Caloric Intake

Enteral tube feedings can also be ordered by calories rather than strength. The physician determines the number of calories the patient requires per day and prescribes prepackaged enteral food feeding. You must determine the amount of the prepackaged enteral food feeding to administer to the patient.

The prepackaged enteral food feeding label specifies the number of calories per volume. You use this information along with the physician's order to calculate the volume of the enteral food feeding to give to your patient.

CALCULATING USING THE ENTERAL TUBE FEEDING FORMULA BY CALORIC INTAKE

Say the physician determined that the patient requires 2000 cal/day and orders that the patient receives Jevity as enteral tube feeding. The label on a can of Jevity states there are 300 cal in every 8 oz. You calculate the number of ounces of Jevity to administer to your patient by using the following formula:

1. Calories = calories/volume of prepackaged external tube feeding
2. Total number of ounces = calories ordered/calories/ounce

Let's apply the formula to the previous example:

1. 35 cal/oz = 280 cal/8 oz
2. 57 oz/day = 2000 cal per day/35 cal/oz

HINT *Remember that 30 mL = 1 oz. You can convert ounces to milliliters if the volume you are administering is in milliliters.*

Practice Drill 9.2—the Enteral Tube Feeding Formula by Calories

Calculate the following enteral tube feedings:

1. The physician ordered that the patient receive 2500 cal/day. You have a 12-oz can of Sustacal. There are 250 cal in 8 oz of Sustacal. How many ounces of Sustacal will the patient receive each day?

2. The physician ordered that the patient receive 2000 cal/day. You have a 12-oz can of Jevity. There are 250 cal in 8 oz of Jevity. How many milliliters will the patient receive each day?

3. The physician ordered that the patient receive 2500 cal/day in 2-hour feedings. You have an 8-oz can of Jevity. There are 350 cal in 8 oz of Jevity. How many ounces will the patient receive in each feeding?

4. The physician ordered that the patient receive 2000 cal/day in 2-hour feedings. You have an 8-oz can of Enrich. There are 200 cal in 8 oz of Enrich. How many milliliters will the patient receive in each feeding?

5. The physician ordered that the patient receive 2500 cal/day in 4-hour feedings. You have a 240-mL can of Enrich. There are 250 cal in 8 oz of Enrich. How many milliliters will the patient receive in each day?

6. The physician ordered that the patient receive 3100 cal/day feedings in 2-hour feedings. You have a 240-mL can of Sustacal. There are 250 cal in 8 oz of Sustacal. How many calories will the patient receive in each feeding?

7. The physician ordered that the patient receive 1800 cal/day feedings. You have an 8-oz can of Sustacal. There are 150 cal in 8 oz of Sustacal. How many cans of Sustacal will the patient receive each day?

8. The physician ordered that the patient receive 2800 cal/day feedings. You have an 8-oz can of Enrich. There are 250 cal in 8 oz of Enrich. How many cans of Enrich will the patient receive each day?

9. The physician ordered that the patient receive 2500 cal/day feedings. You have a 12-oz can of Enrich. There are 150 cal in 8 oz of Enrich. How many cans of Enrich will the patient receive each day?

10. The physician ordered that the patient receive 3500 cal/day feedings in 2-hours feedings. You have a 12-oz can of Jevity. There are 250 cal in 8 oz of Jevity. How many cans of Jevity will the patient receive each day?

Solutions to Practice Drill 9.2—the Enteral Tube Feedings Formula by Caloric Intake

1. 31.25 cal/oz = 250 cal/8 oz.
   80 oz/day = 2500 cal/31.25 cal/oz

2. 31.25 cal/oz = 250 cal/8 oz.
   64 oz = 2000 cal/31.25 cal/oz
   1920 mL/day = 64 oz × 30 mL

3. 43.75 cal/oz = 350 cal/8 oz.
   57.1 oz/day = 2500 cal/43.75 cal/oz
   12 feedings/day = 24 hr/2 hr per feeding
   4.8 oz/feeding = 57.1 oz/day/12 feedings/day

4. 25 cal/oz = 200 cal/8 oz.
   80 oz/day = 2000 cal/25 cal/oz
   12 feedings/day = 24 hr/2 hr per feeding
   6.7 oz/feeding = 80 oz/day/12 feedings/day
   201 mL/feeding = 6.7 oz/feeding × 30 mL

5. 31.25 cal/oz = 250 cal/8 oz.
   80 oz/day = 2500 cal/31.25 cal/oz
   2400 mL/day = 80 oz × 30 mL

6. 12 feedings/day = 24 hr/2 hr per feeding
   258.3 cal/feeding = 3100 calories per day / 12 feedings/day

7. 18.75 cal/oz = 150 cal/8 oz.
   96 oz/day = 1800 cal/18.75 cal/oz
   12 cans per day = 96 oz/day/8 oz

8. 31.25 cal/oz = 250 cal/8 oz.
   89.6 oz/day = 2800 cal/31.25 cal/oz
   11.2 cans per day = 89.6 oz/day/8 oz

9. 18.75 cal/oz = 150 cal/8 oz.
   133.3 oz/day = 2500 cal/18.75 cal/oz
   11.1 cans per day = 133.3 oz/day/12 oz

10. 31.25 cal/oz = 250 cal/8 oz.
    112 oz/day = 3500 cal/31.25 cal/oz
    9.3 cans per day = 112 oz/day/12 oz

Summary

Patients who have difficulty swallowing and who are risk for aspiration are fed through a feeding tube that is either inserted through their nares (NG tube) or surgically inserted into their stomach (PEG) tube. This is referred to as enteral tube feeding.

Although some patients are fed nutrients specifically blended for their needs, many patients are given prepackaged nutrients such as Jevity, Enrich, or Sustacal. These products are at 100% strength.

Physicians might prescribe prepackaged nutrients that are less than 100% strength. This requires you to dilute the prepackaged nutrients with water to arrive at the prescribed strength. The enteral tube feeding formula is used to calculate the amount of water needed to dilute the prepackaged nutrients to arrive at the strength prescribed by the physician.

Alternatively, a physician may prescribe enteral tube feeding by caloric intake. In doing so, the physician specifies total daily calories for the patient and you must determine the amount of the prepackaged nutrients to administer that will give the patient the prescribed caloric intake. You determine this by using the enteral tube feeding formula by caloric intake.

Quiz

1. The physician ordered that the patient receive 2100 cal/day. You have a 12-oz can of Jevity. There are 125 cal in 8 oz of Jevity. How many milliliters will the patient receive each day?

    a. 40.8 mL

    b. 403.8 mL

    c. 4032 mL

    d. 40.38 mL

2. The physician ordered 200 cc of 2/3 strength Jevity via a NG tube. On hand is a 250-cc can of Jevity, which is at 100% strength. How much water is needed to dilute Jevity?

    a. 231 mL

    b. 125 mL

    c. 312 mL

    d. 212 mL

3. The physician ordered 260 cc of 3/4 strength Enrich via a PEG tube. On hand is a 340-cc can of Enrich, which is at full strength. How much water is needed to dilute Enrich?

    a. 120 mL

    b. 119 mL

    c. 123 mL

    d. 113 mL

4. The physician ordered 240 cc of 2/5 strength Sustacal via a PEG tube. On hand is a 210-cc can of Sustacal, which is at full strength. How much water is needed to dilute Sustacal?

   a. 318 mL

   b. 314 mL

   c. 315 mL

   d. 300 mL

5. The physician ordered that the patient receive 3200 cal/day feedings in 2 hour feedings. You have a 240-ml can of Sustacal. There are 225 cal in 8 oz of Sustacal. How many calories will the patient receive in each feeding?

   a. 266.7 cal/feeding

   b. 26.67 cal/feeding

   c. 2.6 cal/feeding

   d. 66.7 cal/feeding

6. The physician ordered 280 cc of 1/4 strength Enrich via a PEG tube. On hand is a 140-mL can of Enrich, which is at full strength. How much water is needed to dilute Enrich?

   a. 420 mL

   b. 400 mL

   c. 415 mL

   d. 404 mL

7. The physician ordered 360 cc of 4/5 strength Enrich via a PEG tube. On hand is a 280-cc can of Enrich, which is at full strength. How much water is needed to dilute Enrich?

   a. 69 mL

   b. 75 mL

   c. 70 mL

   d. 74 mL

8. The physician ordered that the patient receive 2000 calories/day. You have a 12-oz can of Enrich. There are 275 cal in 8 oz of Enrich. How many cans of Enrich will the patient receive each day?

   a. 4.8 cans

   b. 4.7 cans

   c. 4 cans

   d. 4.9 cans

9. The physician ordered 100 cc of 1/5 strength Sustacal via a PEG tube. On hand is a 120-cc can of Sustacal, which is at full strength. How much water is needed to dilute Sustacal?

   a.   450 mL

   b.   480 mL

   c.   400 ml

   d.   350 mL

10. The physician ordered that the patient receive 2200 cal/day. You have a 12-oz can of Sustacal. There are 220 cal in 8 oz of Sustacal. How many cans of Sustacal will the patient receive each day?

   a.   6 cans/day

   b.   6.9 cans/day

   c.   6.6 cans/day

   d.   6.7 cans/day

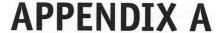

APPENDIX A

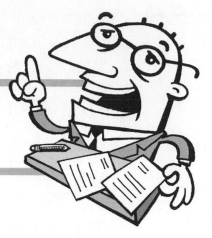

Answering Tricky Questions

All dose calculation questions that you'll be asked on a test can be solved using formulas learned in this book or by using basic math that you learned in grammar school. However, some questions are purposely written to confuse you. Unfair!

Maybe, but the goal is to test your critical thinking skills because in the real world dose calculation problems aren't always presented to you in a clear, concise format. Instead you might be given a bunch of values and you have to pick out those values that you need to calculate your patient's dose.

In this chapter, you'll see tricky questions that are similar to those that you find on tests and you'll learn ways of solving those questions.

Too Many Numbers

You are bound to encounter a question that is purposely designed to confuse you by providing more information than you need to answer the question. The challenge is to select the correct formula and values from the clutter of information in the question.

Here's an example:

Your patient's serum potassium level has been declining. The latest lab shows a serum potassium level of 3.5. Although this is at the low end of the normal range, the physician writes an order for 30 mEq of potassium chloride to be added to 1000 mL of normal saline and administered to your patient over 12 hours. The pharmacy delivers 40 mEq of potassium chloride per 20 mL. How many milliliters of potassium chloride will you administer to your patient?

Probably the first two pieces of information that pop out are 1000 mL and 12 hours. Isn't there a formula that requires converting hours to minutes then divide minutes into milliliters?

Sure there is. But is that the formula needed to answer this question? No. The formula that uses these values calculates the pump setting, which is not what you are asked to calculate. These values are distracters designed to stress you. The information looks like it should be used in the calculation, but you're not sure how to use it—and that's because the information doesn't help you answer the question.

The next two pieces of information that grab your attention are 30 mEq and 1000 mL. Do you divide 30 mEq into 1000 mL? Unsure? This too is a distraction designed to mislead you from the values you really need for the calculation. Why would you divide 30 mEq into 1000 mL? If you can't answer this question, then you are probably on the wrong track.

The question is how many milliliters of potassium chloride will you administer to your patient? The pharmacy delivers 40 mEq of potassium chloride per 20 mL. This is what you have on hand, so you know this must be a component of your calculation. If so, then what did the physician order? 30 mEq potassium chloride. You picked out from the problem the amount ordered and the amount on hand. A bell should sound in your head reminding you of a formula that uses these values.

$$15 \text{ mL} = \frac{30 \text{ mEq}}{40 \text{ mEq}} \times 20 \text{ mL}$$

The Sleight of Hand

Another type of question that you must be prepared to handle is a question whose solution doesn't seem to fit any of the formulas that you are learned. It leaves you scratching your head saying, why should they ask such a dumb question. Whether the question is dumb or not, you must calculate the results that the question poses.

Here's an example:

How many hours does it take for 2 L of normal saline to infuse if the physician writes an order to infuse 2000 mL of normal saline at 125 mL/hr?

At first glance you may say, who cares? If the physician set the amount (1000 mL) and rate (125 mL per hour), then simply set the pump to 125 mL. This is correct if the question was asking you for the pump setting, but it isn't. Knowing the amount of time the drug is infusing helps the nurse in many ways including scheduling activities with that patient and other patients who are assigned to the nurse.

Again, there are more values in the question then you need to calculate the answer. The clue to answering this question is finding the common value. You are asked how many hours to infuse 2 L. You are told that 125 mL is infused each hour. Both specify time and volume.

There are two pieces of information (stressors) in this question that are designed to confuse you. First is 2000 mL ordered by the physician. This doesn't help you solve the problem. And then there is 2 L of normal saline. If you are rushing to answer this question you might overlook the need to calculate common units of measurement. 2 L refers to 2 liters. The physician's order states mL—milliliters.

Once you convert 2 L to milliliters, you'll quickly notice a similarity to the value ordered by the physician:

$$2000 \text{ mL} = 2 \text{ L} \times 1000$$

You can restate the question:

I have 2000 mL infusing at 125 mL/hr. How many hours will this take?

You won't find a formula in this book or probably any book to solve this problem because the solution requires simple division.

$$16 \text{ hours} = \frac{2000 \text{ mL}}{125 \text{ mL}}$$

HINT *If you are asked a question that doesn't seem to be answered by using a dose calculation formula, then think carefully of what you are being asked and then try solving the problem using basic math that you already know.*

The Double Barrel Question

Be alert for a question that asks you two questions in one. You'll be asked to calculate the dose of two different medications that are to be administered to your patient. The objective is to test your critical thinking ability.

Here's the trick to answering the question:

- Identify the two questions that you're being asked to answer.
- Create two columns—one for each drug that you'll be administering according to the question.
- Label the columns with the name of the drug.
- Enter values from the question that pertains to the drug in the corresponding column—be sure to label each value (i.e., ordered and on hand).
- Calculate the dose for each drug—remember that values to calculate the dose of one drug have nothing to do with calculating the dose of the other drug.

The Per Dose Question

Some questions are written to test your thinking skills in addition to your ability to calculate the proper dose to administer to your patient. Here's a typical question that you might be asked on a test:

A young patient who weighs 30 lb has an infection and the physician wants you to administer Ampicillin. The physician's order reads Ampicillin 50 mg/kg per p.o. day for 7 days. The pharmacy delivers 100 mg/mL. The daily dose is given every 6 hours. What dose would you administer to your patient every 6 hours?

There is a lot of information in this question, some of which can be misleading unless you read the question carefully. Here are the tricky parts of this question.

The values represent a daily dose—not a single dose you administer to your patient.

You don't divide the daily dose by 6. There are 4 not 6 doses/day.

It is obvious from the question that you use the pediatric formula. Just remember that the result is for the entire day.

$$13.636 \text{ kg} = \frac{30 \text{ lb}}{2.2 \text{ lb}}$$

$$6.818 \text{ mL/day} = \frac{50 \text{ mg} \times 13.636}{100 \text{ mg}} \times 1 \text{ mL}$$

$$1.7 \text{ mL/dose} = \frac{6.818 \text{ mL}}{4 \text{ doses}}$$

HINT Don't assume that values given in a question pertain to a single dose.

APPENDIX B

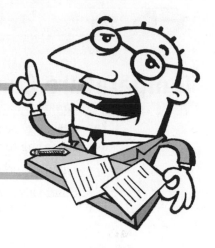

Quick Reference

Conversion Factors

1 mg = 1000 mcg

1 kg = 2.2 lb

1 g = 60 mg

1/100 gr = 0/6 mg

1 in = 2/5 cm

1 cm = 1 mm

1 m = 100 cm

1/150 g = 0/4 mg

1 tsp = 5 mL

1 tbsp = 15 mL

1 oz = 30 mL

1 mmHg = 1.36 cm H20

Temperature Conversion Table

Fahrenheit	Celsius
89.6	32
91.4	33
93.2	34
95.0	35
96.8	36
98.6	37
100.4	38
102.2	39
104.2	40
105.8	41

Temperature Conversion Formulas

$$\text{Celsius} = (\text{Fahrenheit} - 32) \times 0.5555$$
$$\text{Fahrenheit} = (\text{Celcius} \times 1.8) + 32$$

Medication Formulas

INTRAVENOUS DRIP RATE

$$X \text{ gtt/min} = \frac{\text{volume ordered} \times \text{drip factor}}{\text{minutes to infuse}}$$

PUMP RATE

$$\text{Pump rate (mL/hr)} = \frac{\text{volume (mL)}}{\text{time (hr)}}$$

HOW MUCH LONGER WILL THE INTRAVENOUS RUN?

$$\text{Time remaining} = \frac{\text{current volume (mL)}}{\text{pump setting (mL)}}$$

MEDICATION CONCENTRATION

$$\text{Concentration} = \frac{\text{drug quantity (g, mg, mcg)}}{\text{volume of solution (mL)}}$$

DOSE CALCULATION

$$\text{Dose} = \frac{\text{ordered}}{\text{on hand}} \times \text{quantity}$$

WEIGHT-BASED CALCULATION

$$\text{Dose} = \frac{\text{orders (kg)} \times \text{patient's weight (kg)}}{\text{on hand}} \times \text{quantity on hand}$$

MULTI-DOSE FORMULA

$$\text{Dose per day} = \frac{\text{orders (kg)} \times \text{patients's weight (kg)}}{\text{on hand}} \times \text{quantity on hand}$$

$$\text{Dose} = \frac{\text{dose per day}}{\text{ordered number of doses}}$$

HEPARIN CALCULATION MILLILITERS/HOUR

1. Calculate the number of heparin units in a milliliter.

$$\text{Heparin (U/mL)} = \frac{\text{on hand heparin (U)}}{\text{on hand (mL)}}$$

2. Calculate the number of milliliters to administer per hour.

$$\text{Dose (mL/hr)} = \frac{\text{ordered heparin (U)}}{\text{heparin (U/mL)}}$$

HEPARIN CALCULATION IN UNITS

$$\text{Heparin (U/mL)} = \frac{\text{ordered (U)}}{\text{ordered (mL)}}$$

$$\text{Heparin (U)} = \text{heparin (U/mL)} \times \text{ordered (mL/hr)}$$

HEPARIN SUBCUTANEOUS FORMULA

$$\text{Dose} = \frac{\text{ordered}}{\text{on hand}} \times \text{quantity}$$

DOPAMINE FORMULA

1. Convert the patient's weight from pounds to kilograms.

$$\text{Weight (kg)} = \frac{\text{weight (lb)}}{2.2}$$

2. Calculate the concentration of dopamine that is delivered from the pharmacy.

$$\text{Concentration} = \frac{\text{on hand (mg)}}{\text{on hand (mL)}}$$

BODY SURFACE AREA CHILD DOSE CALCULATION FORMULA

$$\text{Child dose} = \frac{\text{body surface area (m}^2)}{1.73 \text{ m}^2} \times \text{adult dose}$$

ENTERAL FOOD FEEDING DILUTION FORMULA

1. Total volume = concentration volume/dilution factor
2. Water to add = total volume − concentration volume

Final Exam—Part 1

1. The physician ordered 1000 mL of 0.9% of sodium chloride I.V. over 60 mL/hr. On hand is tubing with a 10 gtt/mL drip factor. What drip rate would you use?

2. The physician ordered Quinidine Sulfate 400 mg P.O. daily. The pharmacy delivers Quinidine Sulfate 0.2 g per tablet. How many tablets would you administer to your patient?

3. The physician ordered heparin 5250 U s.c. daily. The medication label reads 15,000 U heparin/5 mL. How many milliliters will you administer to the patient per hour?

   a. 1.25 mL

   b. 1 mL

   c. 1.75 mL

   d. 2 mL

   $$\frac{15000}{5\,mL} \times \frac{5250}{x}$$

   $$\frac{15000\,x}{15000} = \frac{26250}{15000}$$

   $$= 1500\overline{)26025.}^{1.0}$$
   $$\underline{-1500}$$
   $$11,250$$

4. The physician ordered Lithostat 120 mg/kg · day q4h. Your patient weighs 110 lb. The pharmacy delivers Lithostat 250 mg/mL. How many milliliters per dose will you administer to your patient?

5. The physician ordered dopamine 7 mcg/kg·min for a patient who weighs 190 lb. The pharmacy delivers dopamine 800 mg in 500 D5W. How many milliliters will you administer to your patient per hour?

6. The physician orders for Vistaril 25 mg and the pharmacy delivered Vistaril 50 mg/mL. What dose would you administer to the patient?

   a. 2 mL

   b. 1.5 mL

   c. 1.0 mL

   d. 0.5 mL

7. The physician ordered 1500 mL normal saline I.V. over 12 hours. What pump setting would you use?

8. The physician ordered Zovirax 10 mg/kg q6h. The patient weighs 77 lb. The medication label reads 100 mg/mL. What dose will you administer to your patient?

   a. 3.5 mL

   b. 3 mL

   c. 4 mL

   d. 4.3 mL

9. The physician ordered dopamine 7 mcg/kg·min for a patient who weighs 155 lb. The pharmacy delivers dopamine 800 mg in 500 D5W. How many milliliters will you administer to your patient per hour?

10. The physician orders for 3000 mL of 1/2 normal saline I.V. that is to be administered over 24 hours. What pump setting will you use?

    a. 124 mL/hr

    b. 120 mL/hr

    c. 125 mL/hr

    d. 126 mL/hr

11. The physician ordered water 1 gal P.O. daily. The patient has an 8-oz cup available at home. How many cups of water should the patient take?

12. The physician ordered 800 mL 1/2 normal saline I.V. over 16 hours. What pump setting will you use?

13. The physician ordered. Dilantin 1 mg/kg q6h. The patient weighs 66 lb. The pharmacy delivers Dilantin 15 mg/1 capsule. How many capsule(s) should you administered to your patient?

14. The physician ordered Benadryl 10 mg/kg q6h. The patient weighs 26 lb. The pharmacy delivers Benadryl 125 mg/5 mL. How many milliliters should you administer to your patient?

15. The physician ordered heparin 400 U/hr. The pharmacy delivers 20,000 U heparin in 2000 mL normal saline. How many milliliters will you administer to your patient per hour?

16. The physician ordered dopamine 5 mcg/kg · min for a patient who weighs 185 lb. The pharmacy delivers dopamine 400 mg in 250 D5W. How many milliliters will you administer to the patient per hour?

17. The physician ordered heparin 800 U/hr. The medication label reads 25,000 U heparin in 250 mL D5W. How many milliliters will you administer to your patient per hour?

    a. 7.5 mL

    b. 7 mL

    c. 8 mL

    d. 8.5 mL

18. The physician ordered Zofran 120 mg/kg I.V. q4h. The patient weighs 33 lb. The medication label reads 200 mg/mL. You will administer 9 mL to the patient.

    a. True

    b. False

19. The physician ordered Xanax 0.25 mg P.O. daily. The pharmacy delivers Xanax 0.5 mg per tablet. How many tablets to administer to the patient?

20. The physician ordered heparin 400 U/hr. The medication label reads 20,000 U heparin in 400 mL normal saline. How many milliliters will you administer to the patient per hour?

    a. 15 mL

    b. 10 mL

    c. 14 mL

    d. 8 mL

21. The physician ordered Erythromycin 100 mg I.V. q6h. The pharmacy delivers Erythromycin 1g/30 mL. How many milliliters will you administer to the patient?

22. The medication order is for 1 L of normal saline I.V. that is to be administered over 8 hours. On hand is I.V. tubing with a 10 gtt/mL drip factor. What is the drip setting?

a. 21 gtt/min

   b. 2.1 gtt/min

   c. 210 gtt/min

23. The physician ordered 350 mL D5W I.V. over 4 hours. What pump setting will you use?

24. The physician ordered Ampicillin 12.5 mg/kg q6h. The patient weighs 40 lb. The pharmacy delivers Ampicillin 100 mg/1 mL. How many milliliters will you administer to the patient?

25. The physician ordered heparin 3000 U s.c. daily. The pharmacy delivers 15,000 U heparin/5 mL. How many milliliters will you administer to the patient?

26. The physician ordered dopamine 6 mcg/kg · min for a patient that weighs 154 lb. The pharmacy delivers dopamine 800 mg in 500 D5W. How many milliliters per hour will you set the infusion pump to?

   a. 15 mL

   b. 16 mL

   c. 14 mL

   d. 17 mL

27. The physician ordered 1 L normal saline I.V. over 12 hours. Use tubing with a 10 gtt/mL drip factor. What is the drip rate?

28. Your patient has received 250 mL of normal saline I.V. and the I.V. bag currently has a volume of 75 mL of normal saline. The pump is set at 30 mL/hr. How much longer does the infusion have to run?

   a. 2 hours 35 minutes

   b. 30 minutes

   c. 2 hours

   d. 2 hours 30 minutes

29. The physician ordered Allopurinol 300 mg P.O. daily. The pharmacy delivers Allopurinol 100 mg per tablet. How many tablets to administer to the patient?

30. The physician ordered 500 mL Ringers Lactate I.V. over 6 hours. Use tubing with a 10 gtt/mL drip factor. What is the drip rate?

31. The physician ordered Benadryl 30 mg/kg · day q6h. The patient weighs 66 lb. The pharmacy delivers Benadryl 125 mg/5 mL. How many milliliters per dose will you administer to the patient?

32. The physician ordered heparin 75 U/hr. The pharmacy delivers 25,000 U heparin in 2000 mL normal saline. How many milliliters will you administer to the patient per hour?

33. The physician ordered heparin 300 U/hr. The pharmacy delivers 20,000 U heparin in 1000 mL D5W. How many milliliters will you administer to the patient per hour?

34. The physician ordered dopamine 3 mcg/kg·min for a patient who weighs 172 lb. The pharmacy delivers dopamine 400 mg in 250 D5W. How many milliliters will you administer to the patient per hour?

35. The physician ordered dopamine 5 mcg/kg·min for a patient who weighs 200 lb. The pharmacy delivers dopamine 800 mg in 500 D5W. How many milliliters will you administer to the patient per hour?

36. The physician ordered Corophyllin 500 mg q6h PRN. The pharmacy delivers Corophyllin 250 mg/1 rectal suppository. How many suppositories will you administer to the patient?

37. The physician ordered Colace 50 mg P.O. daily. The pharmacy delivers Colace 100 mg per tablet. How many milliliters tablets to administer to the patient?

38. The physician ordered Ampicillin 5 mg/kg q6h. The patient weighs 55 lb. The medication label reads 25 mg/mL. What dose will you administer to the patient?

    a.   0.5 mL

    b.   5 mL

    c.   50 mL

    d.   0.05 mL

39. The physician ordered Dilantin 30 mg/kg·day q8h. The patient weighs 55 lb. The pharmacy delivers Dilantin 40 mg/mL. How many milliliters per dose will you administer to the patient?

40. The physician ordered Amoxicillin 10 mg/kg·day q6h. The patient weighs 44 lb. The pharmacy delivers Amoxicillin 125 mg/5 mL. How many milliliters per dose will you administer to the patient?

41. The medication order is for Dilantin 50 mg q6h and the pharmacy delivered Dilantin 125 mg/5 mL. What dose would you administer to the patient?

    a.   5 mL

    b.   4 mL

    c.   3 mL

    d.   2 mL

42. The physician ordered Gentamycin 2 gm diluted in 100 mL of normal saline I.V. over 1 hr. Use tubing with a 15 gtt/mL drip factor. What is the drip rate?

43. The physician ordered 100 mL normal saline I.V. over 15 hours. Use tubing with a 15 gtt/mL drip factor. What is the drip rate?

44. The physician ordered Amoxicillin 10 mg/kg q6h. The patient weighs 30 lb. The pharmacy delivers Amoxicillin 125 mg/5 mL. How many milliliters will you administer to the patient?

45. The physician ordered Celocin 6.25 mg/kg q6h. The patient weighs 45 lb. The pharmacy delivers Celocin 75 mg/5 mL. How many milliliters will you administer to the patient?

46. The physician ordered heparin 600 U/hr. The pharmacy delivers 20,000 U heparin in 1000 mL normal saline. How many milliliters will you administer to the patient per hour?

47. The physician ordered heparin 200 U/hr. The medication label reads 20,000 U heparin in 200 mL normal saline. You will administer 2 mL to patient per hour.

    a. True

    b. False

48. The physician ordered dopamine 5 mcg/kg · min for a patient who weighs 187 lb. The pharmacy delivers dopamine 400 mg in 250 D5W. The infusion pump should be set to 15 mL/hour.

    a. True

    b. False

49. The physician ordered dopamine 5 mcg/kg · min for a patient who weighs 175 lb. The pharmacy delivers dopamine 400 mg in 250 D5W. How many milliliters will you administer to the patient per hour?

50. The physician ordered dopamine 7 mcg/kg · min for a patient who weighs 190 lb. The pharmacy delivers dopamine 800 mg in 500 D5W. How many milliliters will you administer to the patient per hour?

51. The physician ordered 25 mL normal saline I.V. over 30 minutes. Use tubing with a 15 gtt/mL drip factor. What is the drip rate?

52. The physician ordered 1000 mL Ringers Lactate I.V. over 12 hours. Use tubing with 15 gtt/mL drip factor. What is the drip rate?

53. The physician ordered Benylin 5 mg/kg P.O. daily. The patient weighs 44 lb. The pharmacy delivers Benylin 50 mg per tablet. How many tablets will you administer to the patient?

54. The physician ordered Lithostat 15 mg/kg P.O. daily. The patient weighs 70 lb. The pharmacy delivers Lithostat 250 mg per tablet. How many tablets will you administer to the patient?

55. The physician ordered Ampicillin 15 mg/kg · day P.O. q8h. The patient weighs 44 lb. The pharmacy delivers Ampicillin 100 mg/mL. How many milliliters per dose will you administer to the patient?

56. The physician ordered Zofran 120 mg/kg · day q6h. The patient weighs 33 lb. The pharmacy delivers Zofran 200 mg/mL. How many milliliters per dose will you administer to the patient?

57. The physician ordered Lithostat 15 mg/kg I.V. daily. The patient weighs 44 lb. The medication label reads 100 mg/mL. What dose will you administer to the patient?

    a. 5 mL

    b. 4 mL

    c. 3 mL

    d. 2 mL

58. The physician ordered Celocin 10 mg/kg · day q6h. The patient weighs 44 lb. The medication label reads 125mg/5 mL. What dose will you administer to the patient?

    a. 5 mL

    b. 2 mL

    c. 4 mL

    d. 3 mL

59. The medication order is for Cefadyl 10 g diluted in 200 mL of normal saline I.V. that is to be administered over 4 hours. On hand is I.V. tubing with a 15 gtt/mL drip factor. What is the drip setting?

    a. 12 gtt/min

    b. 12.5 gtt/min

    c. 13 gtt/min

    d. 13.5 gtt/min

60. The medication order is for 200 mL of D5W I.V. that is to be administered over 4 hours. The nurse should set the pump at 50 mL/hr.

    a. True

    b. False

61. The physician ordered Capoten 6.25 mg P.O. q8h. The pharmacy delivers Capoten 12.5 mg per tablet. How many tablets to administer to the patient?

62. The physician ordered Morphine Sulfate 2 mg I.M. STAT. The pharmacy delivers Morphine Sulfate 10 mg/mL. How many milliliters to administer to the patient?

63. The physician ordered 1000 mL normal saline I.V. at 40 mL/hr. Use tubing with a 15 gtt/mL drip factor. What is the drip rate?

64. The physician ordered 1000 mL D5W I.V. over 24 hours. What pump setting will you use?

65. The physician ordered 200 mL Lactated Ringers I.V. over 5 hours. What pump setting will you use?

66. The physician ordered Zovirax 5 mg/kg I.V. daily. The patient weighs 30 lb. The pharmacy delivers Zovirax 25 mg/mL. What pump setting will you use?

67. The physician ordered Benylin 25 mg/kg·day I.M. q3h. The patient weighs 55 lb. The pharmacy delivers Benylin 25 mg/mL. How many milliliters per dose will you administer to the patient?

68. The physician ordered heparin 200 U/hr. The pharmacy delivers 25,000 U heparin in 500 mL D5W. How many milliliters will you administer to the patient per hour?

69. The physician ordered heparin 250 U/hr. The pharmacy delivers 25,000 U heparin in 1000 mL D5W. How many milliliters will you administer to the patient per hour?

70. The physician ordered heparin 2500 U s.c. The pharmacy delivers 25,000 U heparin/10 mL. How many milliliters will you administer to the patient?

71. The physician ordered heparin 2000 U s.c. The pharmacy delivers 20,000 U heparin/5 mL. How many milliliters will you administer to the patient?

72. The physician ordered dopamine 7 mcg/kg·min for a patient who weighs 240 lb. The pharmacy delivers dopamine 400 mg in 250 D5W. How many milliliters per hour will you set the infusion pump to?

    a. 28 mL

    b. 29 mL

    c. 28.6 mL

    d. 28.63 mL

73. The physician ordered dopamine 3 mcg/kg·min for a patient who weighs 180 lb. The pharmacy delivers dopamine 400 mg in 250 D5W. How many milliliters per hour will you set the infusion pump to?

a. 10 mL

    b. 9.20 mL

    c. 9 mL

    d. 9.2 mL

74. The physician ordered Lopid 0.6 g P.O. daily. The pharmacy delivers Lopid 600 mg per tablet. How many tablets will you administer to the patient?

75. The physician ordered Amphojet 5 mL P.O. daily. The patient has a teaspoon available at home. How many teaspoons of the Amphojet should the patient take?

76. The physician ordered 1500 mL Lactated Ringers I.V. over 16 hours. What pump setting will you use?

77. The physician ordered 150 mL D51/2 normal saline I.V. over 5 hours. What pump setting will you use?

78. The physician ordered Zofran 150 mcg/kg I.M. daily. The patient weighs 65 lb. The pharmacy delivers Zofran 2000 mcg/mL. How many milliliters will you administer to the patient?

79. The physician ordered heparin 800 U/hr. The pharmacy delivers 10,000 U heparin in 500 mL normal saline. How many milliliters will you administer to the patient per hour?

80. The physician ordered heparin 400 U/hr. The pharmacy delivers 25,000 U heparin in 2000 mL D5W. How many milliliters will you administer to the patient per hour?

81. The physician ordered dopamine 8 mcg/kg·min for a patient who weighs 220 lb. The pharmacy delivers dopamine 400 mg in 250 D5W. How many milliliters per hour will you set the infusion pump to?

    a. 30 mL

    b. 29.5 mL

    c. 31 mL

    d. 29 mL

82. The physician ordered dopamine 3 mcg/kg·min for a patient who weighs 132 lb. The pharmacy delivers dopamine 400 mg in 250 D5W. How many milliliters per hour will you set the infusion pump to?

    a. 6 mL

    b. 6.2 mL

    c. 6.5 mL

    d. 6.75 mL

83. The physician ordered heparin 7500 U s.c. The pharmacy delivers 20,000 U heparin/2 mL. How many milliliters will you administer to the patient?

84. The physician ordered heparin 8000 U s.c. The pharmacy delivers 20,000 U heparin/10 mL. How many milliliters will you administer to the patient?

85. The physician ordered heparin 100 U/hr. The medication label reads 20,000 U heparin in 2000 mL D5W. How many milliliters will you administer to the patient per hour?

    a. 1 mL

    b. 1.9 mL

    c. 0.9 mL

    d. 10 mL

86. The physician ordered 500 mL D5 1/2 normal saline I.V. over 8 hours. What pump setting will you use?

87. The physician ordered Zovirax 5mg/kg·day P.O. q12h. The patient weighs 55 lbs. The pharmacy delivers Zovirax 25 mg/tablet. How many tablets per dose will you administer to the patient?

88. The physician ordered Celocin 45 mg/kg·day P.O. q4h. The patient weighs 110 lb. The pharmacy delivers Celocin 125 mg/5 mL. How many milliliters per dose will you administer to the patient?

89. The physician ordered Cephalexin 15 mg/kg·day P.O. q6h. The patient weighs 132 lb. The pharmacy delivers Cephalexin 125 mg/5 mL. How many milliliters per dose will you administer to the patient?

90. The physician ordered heparin 5000 U s.c. The pharmacy delivers 20,000 U heparin/2 mL. How many milliliters will you administer to the patient?

91. The physician ordered heparin 4000 U s.c. The pharmacy delivers 10,000 U heparin/mL. How many milliliters will you administer to the patient?

92. The physician ordered dopamine 8 mcg/kg·min for a patient who weighs 165 lb. The pharmacy delivers dopamine 400 mg in 250 D5W. How many milliliters will you administer to the patient per hour?

93. The physician ordered dopamine 4 mcg/kg·min for a patient who weighs 184 lb. The pharmacy delivers dopamine 400 mg in 250 D5W. How many milliliters will you administer to the patient per hour?

94. The medication order is for Motrin 0.6 g P.O. q6h and the pharmacy delivered Motrin 400 mg per tablet. What dose would you administer to the patient?

    a. 1 tablet

    b. 1.25 tablets

c. 1.5 tablets

    d. 0.5 tablet

95. The medication order is for Decadron 3 mg P.O. q6h and the pharmacy delivered Decadron 0.75 mg per tablet. What dose would you administer to the patient?

    a. 2.5 tablets

    b. 2 tablets

    c. 4 tablets

    d. 4.5 tablets

96. The physician ordered Methozamine HCl 0.015 g I.M. daily. The pharmacy delivers Methozamine HCl 10 mg/mL. How many milliliters will you administer to the patient?

97. The physician ordered Milk of Magnesia 30 mL P.O. daily. The patient has a tablespoon available at home. How many tablespoons should the patient take of Milk of Magnesia?

98. The physician ordered fruit juice 4000 mL P.O. daily. The patient has a 1-qt container available at home. How many quarts should the patient take of fruit juice?

99. The medication order is for 600 mL of 1/2 normal saline I.V. that is to be administered over 6 hours. On hand is I.V. tubing with a 10 gtt/mL drip factor. What pump setting will you use?

    a. 15 gtt/min

    b. 16 gtt/min

    c. 17 gtt/min

    d. 18 gtt/min

100. The physician ordered Cephalexin 15 mg/kg P.O. daily. The patient weighs 45 lb. The pharmacy delivers Cephalexin 125 mg/5 mL. How many milliliters will you administer to the patient?

Final Exam—Part 2

1. The medication order is for 2 L of normal saline I.V. that is to be administered over 16 hours. On hand is I.V. tubing with a 15 gtt/mL drip factor. What is the drip setting?

   a.   31 gtt/min

   b.   3.1 gtt/min

   c.   310 gtt/min

2. The medication order is for Dilantin 75 mg and the pharmacy delivered Dilantin 150 mg/2 mL. What dose would you administer to the patient?

   a.   2 mL

   b.   1.5 mL

   c.   1 mL

   d.   2.5 mL

3. Your patient has received 500 mL of sodium chloride I.V. and the I.V. bag currently has a volume of 50 mL of sodium chloride. The pump is set at 20 mL/hr. How much longer does the infusion have to run?

a. 2 hours 5 minutes

    b. 30 minutes

    c. 2 hours

    d. 2 hours 30 minutes

4. The physician ordered 500 mL Ringers Lactate I.V. over 24 hours. Use microdrip tubing. What is the drip rate?

5. The physician ordered Erythromycin 200 mg I.V. The pharmacy delivers Erythromycin 2g/60 mL. How many milliliters will you administer to the patient?

6. The physician ordered dopamine 5 mcg/kg · min for a patient who weighs 125 lb. The pharmacy delivers dopamine 800 mg in 500 D5W. How many milliliters will you administer to your patient per hour?

7. The physician ordered dopamine 6 mcg/kg · min for a patient who weighs 150 lb. The pharmacy delivers dopamine 800 mg in 500 D5W. How many milliliters will you administer to the patient per hour?

8. The medication order is for Cefadyl 50 gm diluted in 300 mL of normal saline I.V. that is to be administered over 8 hours. On hand is I.V. tubing with a 10 gtt/mL drip factor. What is the drip setting?

    a. 6 gtt/min

    b. 6.5 gtt/min

    c. 7 gtt/min

    d. 7.5 gtt/min

9. The physician ordered heparin 4000 U s.c. The pharmacy delivers 20,000 U heparin/150 mL. How many milliliters will you administer to the patient?

10. The physician ordered dopamine 4 mcg/kg · min for a patient who weighs 175 lb. The pharmacy delivers dopamine 800 mg in 500 D5W. How many milliliters will you administer to the patient per hour?

11. The physician ordered Corophyllin 500 mg q8h PRN. The pharmacy delivers Corophyllin 250 mg/rectal suppository. How many rectal suppositories to administer to the patient?

12. The physician ordered Heparin 800 U/hr. The medication label reads 20,000 U heparin in 600 mL normal saline. How many milliliters will you administer to the patient per hour?

    a. 25 mL

    b. 20 mL

    c. 24 mL

    d. 23 mL

13. The physician ordered Ampicillin 20 mg/kg. The patient weighs 157 lb.
    The medication label reads 50 mg/mL. What dose will you administer to
    your patient?

    a. 28.5 mL

    b. 28 mL

    c. 29 mL

    d. 29.5 mL

14. The physician ordered Amoxicillin 30 mg/kg. The patient weighs 66 lb.
    The pharmacy delivers Amoxicillin 250 mg/10 mL. How many milliliters
    will you administer to the patient?

15. The physician ordered dopamine 6 mcg/kg · min for a patient who weighs
    280 lb. The pharmacy delivers dopamine 800 mg in 500 mL D5W. How
    many milliliters per hour will you set the infusion pump?

    a. 27 mL

    b. 27.5 mL

    c. 29 mL

    d. 28.6 mL

16. The physician ordered 150 mL D51/2 normal saline I.V. over 2 hours. What
    pump setting will you use?

17. The physician ordered Milk of Magnesia 15 mL P.O. q.i.d. The patient has a
    tablespoon available at home. How many tablespoons of Milk of Magnesia
    should the patient take?

18. The physician ordered Morphine sulfate 32 mg I.M. STAT. The pharmacy
    delivers Morphine sulfate 15 mg/mL. How many milliliters will you
    administer to the patient?

19. The physician ordered Gentamycin 4 gm diluted in 200 mL of normal
    saline I.V. over 2 hours. Use tubing with a 10 gtt/mL drip factor. What is
    the drip rate?

20. The physician ordered 650 mL D5W I.V. over 8 hours. What pump setting
    will you use?

21. The physician orders are for 250 mL of 1/2 normal saline I.V. that is to be
    administered over 12 hours. What pump setting will you use?

    a. 20.75 mL/hr

    b. 20 mL/hr

    c. 20.8 mL/hr

    d. 20.7 mL/hr

22. The physician ordered 500 mL of 0.9% of normal saline I.V. over 30 mL/hr. On hand is tubing with a15 gtt/mL drip factor. What drip rate would you use?

23. The physician ordered Ampicillin 15 mg/kg. The patient weighs 80 lb. The pharmacy delivers Ampicillin 200 mg/mL. How many milliliters will you administer to the patient?

24. The physician ordered Celocin 3.25 mg/kg. The patient weighs 75 lb. The pharmacy delivers Celocin 50 mg/5 mL. How many milliliters will you administer to the patient?

25. The physician ordered Zofran 140 mg/kg·day q8h. The patient weighs 77 lb. The pharmacy delivers Zofran 250 mg/mL. How many milliliters per dose will you administer to the patient?

26. The physician ordered 2000 mL normal saline I.V. at 20 mL/hr. Use tubing with a 15 gtt/mL drip factor. What is the drip rate?

27. The physician ordered dopamine 5 mcg/kg·min for a patient who weighs 340 lb. The pharmacy delivers dopamine 400 mg in 250 D5W. How many milliliters per hour will you set the infusion pump?

    a. 28 mL

    b. 29 mL

    c. 28.6 mL

    d. 28.63 mL

28. The physician ordered heparin 200 U/hr. The pharmacy delivers 25,000 U heparin in 4000-mL D5W. How many milliliters will you administer to the patient per hour?

29. The physician ordered heparin 4000 U s.c. The pharmacy delivers 25,000 U heparin/800 mL. How many milliliters will you administer to the patient?

30. The physician ordered heparin 600 U/hr. The pharmacy delivers 15,000 U heparin in 500-mL normal saline. How many milliliters will you administer to the patient per hour?

31. The physician ordered Zovirax 2mg/kg·day q12h. The patient weighs 160 lb. The pharmacy delivers Zovirax 50 mg per tablet. How many tablets per dose will you administer to the patient?

32. The physician ordered Benylin 25 mg/kg. The patient weighs 88 lb. The pharmacy delivers Benylin 75 mg per tablet. How many tablets will you administer to the patient?

33. The physician ordered Gentamycin 0.55 mg P.O. q.i.d. The pharmacy delivers Gentamycin 0.75 mg per 2 tablets. How many tablets will you administer to the patient?

34. The physician ordered dopamine 10 mcg/kg·min for a patient who weighs 170 lb. The pharmacy delivers dopamine 800 mg in 500 D5W. How many milliliters will you administer to your patient per hour?

35. The physician ordered Zofran 100 mg/kg. The patient weighs 75 lb. The medication label reads 250 mg/mL. You will administer 15 mL to the patient.

    a. True

    b. False

36. The physician ordered heparin 6000 U s.c. The medication label reads 20,000 U heparin/100 mL. How many milliliters will you administer to the patient per hour?

    a. 30.25 mL

    b. 30 mL

    c. 30.75 mL

    d. 40 mL

37. The physician ordered Benadryl 35 mg/kg·day q12h. The patient weighs 82 lb. The pharmacy delivers Benadryl 250 mg/10 mL. How many milliliters per dose will you administer to the patient?

38. The physician ordered Heparin 25, 000 U/hr. The medication label reads 20,000 U heparin in 3000 mL normal saline. You will administer 5 mL/hr to the patient.

    a. True

    b. False

39. The physician ordered Amphojet 15 mL P.O. q.i.d. The patient has a teaspoon available at home. How many teaspoons will the patient require to administer Amphojet 15 mL?

40. The physician ordered heparin 1000 U s.c. The pharmacy delivers 20,000 U heparin/700 mL. How many milliliters will you administer to the patient?

41. The physician ordered Cephalexin 10 mg/kg. The patient weighs 145 lb. The pharmacy delivers Cephalexin 125 mg/8 mL. How many milliliters will you administer to the patient?

42. The medication order is for 500 mL of D5W I.V. that is to be administered over 8 hours. The nurse should set the pump at 75 mL/hr.

    a. True

    b. False

43. The physician ordered heparin 300 U/hr. The pharmacy delivers 25,000 U heparin in 800 mL D5W. How many milliliters will you administer to the patient per hour?

44. The physician ordered Benylin 15 mg/kg. The patient weighs 30 lb. The pharmacy delivers Benylin 50 mg per tablet. How many tablets will you administer to the patient?

45. The physician ordered Ampicillin 15 mg/kg. The patient weighs 45 lb. The pharmacy delivers Ampicillin 250 mg/10 mL. How many milliliters should you administered to your patient?

46. The physician ordered Dilantin 60 mg/kg·day q4h. The patient weighs 130 lb. The pharmacy delivers Dilantin 125 mg/mL. How many milliliters per dose will you administer to your patient?

47. The physician ordered Ampicillin 75 mg. The patient weighs 95 lb. The medication label reads 50 mg/mL. What dose will you administer to the patient?

    a.   1.5 mL

    b.   0.15 mL

    c.   50 mL

    d.   0.05 mL

48. The physician ordered Celocin 20 mg/kg·day q6h. The patient weighs 125lb. The medication label reads 175 mg/5 mL. What dose will you administer to the patient?

    a.   8.1 mL

    b.   8.2 mL

    c.   8 mL

    d.   7.5 mL

49. The physician ordered heparin 3500 U s.c. The pharmacy delivers 25,000 U heparin/200 mL. How many milliliters will you administer to the patient?

50. The physician ordered heparin 7000 U s.c. The pharmacy delivers 20,000 U heparin/300 mL. How many milliliters will you administer to the patient?

51. The medication order is for Motrin 0.8 g and the pharmacy delivered Motrin 400 mg per tablet. What dose would you administer to the patient?

    a.   1 tablet

    b.   1.25 tablets

    c.   1.5 tablets

    d.   2 tablets

52. The physician ordered Lithostat 6 mg/kg. The patient weighs 150 lb. The pharmacy delivers Lithostat 150 mg per tablet. How many tablets will you administer to the patient?

53. The physician ordered Dilantin 15 mg/kg·day q8h. The patient weighs 150 lb. The pharmacy delivers Dilantin 20 mg/mL. How many milliliters per dose will you administer to the patient?

54. The physician ordered Benadryl 2 mg/kg. The patient weighs 88 lb. The pharmacy delivers Benadryl 25 mg/1 capsule. How many capsule(s) will you administered to the patient?

55. The physician ordered Zovirax 200 mg P.O. q.i.d. The pharmacy delivers Zovirax 0.1 g per tablet. How many tablets would you administer to your patient?

56. The physician ordered dopamine 12 mcg/kg·min for a patient who weighs 170 lb. The pharmacy delivers dopamine 800 mg in 500 D5W. How many milliliters per hour will you set the infusion pump?

    a. 32.2 mL

    b. 30 mL

    c. 34.8 mL

    d. 35 mL

57. The physician ordered Amoxicillin 20 mg/kg·day q6h. The patient weighs 97 lb. The pharmacy delivers Amoxicillin 125 mg/10 mL. How many milliliters per dose will you administer to the patient?

58. The physician ordered Zovirax 8 mg/kg. The patient weighs 45 lb. The pharmacy delivers Zovirax 25 mg/mL. How many milliliters per dose will you administer to the patient?

59. The physician ordered dopamine 2 mcg/kg·min for a patient who weighs 120 lb. The pharmacy delivers dopamine 400 mg in 250 mL D5W. How many milliliters per hour will you set the infusion pump?

60. The physician ordered dopamine 10 mcg/kg·min for a patient who weighs 85 lb. The pharmacy delivers dopamine 400 mg in 250 mL D5W. How many milliliters will you administer to the patient per hour?

61. The physician ordered Benylin 15 mg/kg·day q3h. The patient weighs 75 lb. The pharmacy delivers Benylin 50 mg/1 mL. How many milliliters per dose will you administer to the patient?

62. The physician ordered dopamine 15 mcg/kg·min for a patient that weighs 194 lb. The pharmacy delivers dopamine 800 mg in 500 mL D5W. The infusion pump should be set to 15 mL/hr.

a. True

b. False

63. The physician ordered heparin 500 U/hr. The pharmacy delivers 20, 000 U heparin in 2000-mL D5W. How many milliliters will you administer to the patient per hour?

64. The physician ordered dopamine 35 mcg/kg·min for a patient who weighs 125 lb. The pharmacy delivers dopamine 400 mg in 250 D5W. How many milliliters will you administer to the patient per hour?

65. The physician ordered Capoten 3 mg P.O. q8h. The pharmacy delivers Capoten 6 mg per tablet. How many tablets will you administer to the patient?

66. The physician ordered 250 mL D51/2 normal saline I.V. over 6 hours. What pump setting will you use?

67. The physician ordered dopamine 6 mcg/kg·min for a patient who weighs 284 lb. The pharmacy delivers dopamine 800 mg in 500 D5W. How many milliliters will you administer to the patient per hour?

68. The medication order is for 900 mL of 1/2 normal saline I.V. that is to be administered over 8 hours. On hand is I.V. tubing with a 15 gtt/mL drip factor. What pump setting will you use?

a. 112.5 mL/hr

b. 111 mL/hr

c. 100 mL/hr

d. 112 mL/hr

69. The physician ordered Zofran 250 mcg/kg. The patient weighs 165 lb. The pharmacy delivers Zofran 4000 mcg/mL. How many milliliters will you administer to the patient?

a. 4 mL

b. 4.7 mL

c. 3.7 mL

d. 3 mL

70. The physician ordered Ampicillin 25 mg/kg·day q8h. The patient weighs 65 lb. The pharmacy delivers Ampicillin 125 mg/mL. How many milliliters per dose will you administer to the patient?

71. The physician ordered 750 mL Ringers Lactate I.V. over 18 hour. Use tubing with a 10 gtt/mL drip factor. What is the drip rate?

72. The physician ordered Heparin 1000 U/hr. The medication label reads 25,000 U heparin in 250 mL D5W. How many milliliters will you administer to your patient per hour?

    a.   10 mL

    b.   12 mL

    c.   13 mL

    d.   12.5 mL

73. The physician ordered 250 mL sodium chloride I.V. over 18 hours. What pump setting would you use?

74. The physician ordered Allopurinol 250 mg P.O. q.i.d. The pharmacy delivers Allopurinol 150 mg per 2 tablets. How many tablets to administer to the patient?

75. The physician ordered 50 mL normal saline I.V. over 30 minutes. Use tubing with a 10 gtt/mL drip factor. What is the drip rate?

76. The physician ordered Lopid 0.8 g P.O. q.i.d. The pharmacy delivers Lopid 800 mg per tablet. How many tablets to administer to the patient?

77. The physician ordered Heparin 250 U/hr. The medication label reads 20,000 U heparin in 4000 mL D5W. How many milliliters will you administer to the patient per hour?

    a.   52 mL

    b.   51 mL

    c.   50 mL

    d.   49 mL

78. The medication order is for Decadron 2 mg and the pharmacy delivered Decadron 0.50 mg per tablet. What dose would you administer to the patient?

    a.   2.5 tablets

    b.   2 tablets

    c.   4 tablets

    d.   4.5 tablets

79. The physician ordered 2000 mL D5W I.V. over 16 hours. What pump setting will you use?

80. The physician ordered heparin 800 U/hr. The pharmacy delivers 20,000 U heparin in 2000 mL normal saline. How many milliliters will you administer to the patient per hour?

81. The physician ordered 1600 mL1/2 sodium chloride I.V. over 18 hours. What pump setting will you use?

82. The physician ordered dopamine 9 mcg/kg·min for a patient who weighs 125 lb. The pharmacy delivers dopamine 400 mg in 250 D5W. How many milliliters will you administer to your patient per hour?

83. The physician orders for Xanax 35 mg and the pharmacy delivered Xanax 75 mg/5 mL. What dose would you administer to the patient?

    a. 0.22 mL

    b. 0.25 mL

    c. 0.3 mL

    d. 0 mL

84. The physician ordered 3000 mL normal saline I.V. over 24 hours. Use tubing with a 10 gtt/mL drip factor. What is the drip rate?

85. The physician ordered 2500 mL Lactated Ringers I.V. over 24 hours. What pump setting will you use?

86. The physician ordered Celocin 15 mg/kg·day q8h. The patient weighs 210 lb. The pharmacy delivers Celocin 125 mg/2 mL. How many milliliters per dose will you administer to the patient?

87. The physician ordered fruit juice 2000 mL P.O. q.i.d. The patient has a 1-qt container available at home. How many quarts should the patient take of fruit juice?

88. The physician ordered heparin 800 U s.c. The pharmacy delivers 25,000 U heparin/500 mL. How many milliliters will you administer to the patient?

89. The physician ordered heparin 350 U s.c. The pharmacy delivers 15,000 U heparin/200 mL. How many milliliters will you administer to the patient?

90. The physician ordered heparin 600 U/hr. The pharmacy delivers 15,000 U heparin in 1000 mL normal saline. How many milliliters will you administer to your patient per hour?

91. The physician ordered Colace 400 mg P.O. q.i.d. The pharmacy delivers Colace 200 mg/1 capsule. How many milliliters you will administer to the patient?

92. The physician ordered heparin 500 U/hr. The pharmacy delivers 25,000 U heparin in 2000 mL D5W. How many milliliters will you administer to the patient per hour?

93. The physician ordered dopamine 6 mcg/kg·min for a patient who weighs 232 lb. The pharmacy delivers dopamine 400 mg in 250 D5W. How many milliliters per hour will you set the infusion pump?

a. 23.5 mL

   b. 23 mL

   c. 23.8 mL

   d. 23.7 mL

94. The physician ordered Cephalexin 10 mg/kg·day q8h. The patient weighs 232 lb. The pharmacy delivers Cephalexin 250 mg/5 mL. How many milliliters per dose will you administer to the patient?

95. The physician ordered dopamine 15 mcg/kg·min for a patient who weighs 250 lb. The pharmacy delivers dopamine 800 mg in 500 D5W. How many milliliters will you administer to the patient per hour?

96. The physician ordered Lithostat 5 mg/kg. The patient weighs 85 lb. the medication label reads 150 mg/mL. What dose will you administer to the patient?

   a. 1.55 mL.

   b. 1.4 mL

   c. 1.3 mL

   d. 1.2 mL

97. The physician ordered GoLytely 1 gal P.O. q.i.d. The patient has a 12-oz cup available at home. How many cups of GoLytely should the patient take?

98. The physician ordered 400 mL Lactated Ringers I.V. over 8 hours. What pump setting will you use?

99. The physician ordered heparin 50 U/hr. The pharmacy delivers 25,000 U heparin in 3000 mL normal saline. How many milliliters will you administer to the patient per hour?

100. The physician ordered Methozamine HCl 0.025 g I.M. q.i.d. The pharmacy delivers Methozamine HCl 20 mg/mL. How many milliliters will you administer to the patient?

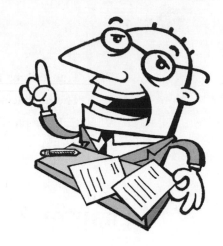

Answers to Quiz and Exam Questions

Chapter 1

1. b. Call the physician
2. c. Call the physician
3. a. Calculate the dose and administer the medication
4. b. False
5. c. Provide instructions to the nurse for when to give the medication
6. b. Immediately after the medication is administered

7. a. Transcribing a medication order to the MAR

8. a. The healthcare facility's policy

9. a. Call the physician

10. a. 01000

Chapter 2

1. a. 2 tablets

2. c. 1.5 tablets

3. c. 4 tablets

4. a. True

5. b. 2 tablets

6. d. 0.5 mL

7. b. 2 capsules

8. a. 2 mL

9. a. 2 tablets

10. c. 0.67 mL

Chapter 3

1. b. 2.5 mL

2. d. 0.5 mL

3. b. 2 tablets

4. a. True

5. a. 1.5 mL

6. c. 4 mL

7. b. 2 capsules

8. c. 2 capsules

9. d. 3.5 tablets

10. c. 5 tablets

Chapter 4

1. b. 200 mL
2. a. 21 gtt/min
3. c. 13 gtt/min
4. a. True
5. d. 2 hours 30 minutes
6. d. 4.8 gtt/min
7. c. 125 mL/hr
8. a. 31 gtt/min
9. a. 100 mL/hr
10. d. 18 hours 45 minutes

Chapter 5

1. a. 4 mL
2. c. 15 mL
3. b. 5 mL
4. a. True
5. c. 3 mL
6. c. 0.4 mL
7. d. 9 mL
8. a. 7.2 mL
9. d. 2.4 mL
10. a. 3.5 mL

Chapter 6

1. c. 5 mL
2. c. 8 mL
3. b. 6 mL

4. a. True
5. c. 1.75 mL
6. b. 8 mL
7. d. 10 mL
8. a. 2.25 mL
9. d. 12 mL
10. a. 20 mL

Chapter 7

1. a. 30 mL
2. d. 6.75 mL
3. b. 16 mL
4. a. True
5. a. 7 mL
6. b. 29 mL
7. b. 9.2 mL
8. a. 13 mL
9. b. 14.6 mL
10. c. 18.3 mL

Chapter 8

1. a. 32.5 mg
2. c. 11.6 mg
3. b. 14.5 mg
4. a. 8.7 mg
5. a. 31.8 mg
6. b. 86.7 mg
7. c. 46.2 mg

8. a. 10.4 mg
9. d. 40.5 mg
10. d. 130 mg

Chapter 9

1. c. 4032 mL
2. b. 125 mL
3. d. 113 mL
4. c. 315 mL
5. a. 266.7 calories/feeding
6. a. 420 mL
7. c. 70 mL
8. a. 4.8 cans
9. b. 480 mL
10. d. 6.7 cans/day

Final Exam—Part 1

1. 10 gtt/min
2. 2 tablets
3. c. 1.75 mL
4. 4 mL
5. 25 mL/hr
6. d. 0.5 mL
7. 125 mL
8. a. 3.5 mL
9. 18.5 mL
10. c. 125 mL/hr
11. 16 cups
12. 50 mL

13. 2 capsules

14. 4.7 mL

15. 40 mL

16. 16 mL/hr

17. c. 8 mL

18. a. True

19. 0.5 tablet

20. d. 8 mL

21. 3 mL

22. a. 21 gtt/min

23. 88 mL

24. 2.3 mL

25. 1 mL

26. b. 16 mL

27. 14 gtt/min

28. d. 2 hours 30 minutes

29. 3 tablet

30. 14 gtt/min

31. 9 mL

32. 6 mL

33. 15 mL

34. 9 mL/hr

35. 17 mL/hr

36. 2 rectal suppositories

37. 0.5 tablet

38. b. 5 mL

39. 6.25 mL

40. 2 mL

41. d. 2 mL

42. 25 gtt/min

43. 10 gtt/min

44. 5.5 mL

45. 8.5 mL
46. 30 mL
47. a. True
48. a. True
49. 15 mL/hr
50. 23 mL/hr
51. 13 gtt/min
52. 21 gtt/min
53. 2 tablets
54. 2 tablets
55. 1 mL
56. 2.25 mL
57. c. 3 mL
58. b. 2 mL
59. c. 13 gtt/min
60. a. True
61. 0.5 tablet
62. 0.2 mL
63. 10 gtt/min
64. 42 mL
65. 40 mL
66. 2.7 mL
67. 3.13 mL
68. 4 mL
69. 1 mL
70. 1 mL
71. 0.5 mL
72. b. 29 mL
73. c. 9 mL
74. 1 tablet
75. 1 teaspoon
76. 94 mL

77. 30 mL

78. 2.2 mL

79. 40 mL

80. 32 mL

81. a. 30 mL

82. d. 6.75 mL

83. 0.75 mL

84. 4 mL

85. d. 10 mL

86. 62.5 mL

87. 2.5 tablets

88. 15 mL

89. 9 mL

90. 0.5 mL

91. 0.4 mL

92. 22.5 mL/hr

93. 12.5 mL/hr

94. c. 1.5 tablets

95. c. 4.0 tablets

96. 1.5 mL

97. 2 tablespoons

98. 4 qt

99. c. 17 gtt/min

100. 12 mL

Final Exam—Part 2

1. a. 31 gtt/min

2. c. 1.0 mL

3. d. 2 hours 30 minutes

4. 21 gtt/min

5. 6 mL

6. 10.7 mL

7. 15.3 mL/hr

8. b. 6.5 gtt/min

9. 30 mL

10. 11.9 mL/hr

11. 2 rectal suppositories

12. c. 24 mL

13. a. 28.5 mL

14. 36 mL

15. d. 28.6 mL

16. 75 mL

17. 1 tablespoon

18. 2.1 mL

19. 7 gtt/min

20. 81.25 mL/hr

21. c. 20.8 mL/hr

22. 8 gtt/min

23. 2.7 mL

24. 11 mL

25. 6.5 mL

26. 5 gtt/min

27. b. 29 mL

28. 32 mL

29. 128 mL

30. 20 mL

31. 1.5 tablets

32. 13 tablets

33. 0.5 tablet

34. 29 mL/hr

35. b. False

36. b. 30 mL

37. 26 mL

38. b. False
39. 3 teaspoons
40. 2 mL
41. 42.2 mL
42. b. False
43. 9.6 mL/hr
44. 4 tablets
45. 12.3 mL
46. 4.7 mL
47. a. 1.5 mL
48. a. 8.1 mL
49. 28 mL
50. 105 mL
51. d. 2 tablets
52. 3 mL
53. 17 mL
54. 3 capsules
55. 2 tablets
56. c. 34.8 mL
57. 17.6 mL
58. 6.5 mL
59. 4.1 mL/hr
60. 14.5 mL/hr
61. 1.3 mL
62. b. False
63. 50 mL/hr
64. 74.6 mL/hr
65. 0.5 tablet
66. 41.7 mL/hr
67. 29 mL/hr
68. a. 112.5 mL/hr
69. b. 4.7 mL

70. 2 mL
71. 6.9 gtt/min
72. a. 10 mL
73. 13.9 mL/hr
74. 3 tablets
75. 17 gtt/min
76. 1 tablet
77. c. 50 mL
78. c. 4 tablets
79. 125 mL/hr
80. 80 mL/hr
81. 88.9 mL/hr
82. 19.2 mL/hr
83. a. 0.22 mL
84. 20.8 gtt/min
85. 104.2 mL/hr
86. 7.6 mL
87. 2 qt
88. 16 mL
89. 4.7 mL
90. 40 mL/hr
91. 2 capsules
92. 40 mL/hr
93. d. 23.7 mL
94. 7 mL
95. 63.9 mL/hr
96. c. 1.3 mL
97. 11 cups
98. 50 mL/hr
99. 6 mL/hr
100. 1.25 mL

INDEX

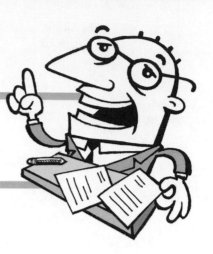

Note: Page numbers referencing figures are italicized and followed by an "*f*". Page numbers referencing tables are italicized and followed by a "*t*".